D1558389

HANDBOOK OF CHROMOSOMAL SYNDROMES

HANDBOOK OF CHROMOSOMAL SYNDROMES

G. Shashidhar Pai, M.D.
Department of Pediatrics
Medical University of South Carolina
Charleston, South Carolina

Raymond C. Lewandowski, Jr., M.D.
Raymond C. Lewandowski, Jr., M.D., P.A.
Corpus Christi, Texas

Digamber S. Borgaonkar, Ph.D.
Retired Director
Cytogenetics Laboratory
Christiana Care Health Systems
Newark, Delaware

Laboratory of Neurogenetics
National Institute of Aging
National Institutes of Health
Bethesda, Maryland

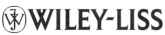WILEY-LISS
A JOHN WILEY & SONS, INC., PUBLICATION

Published by John Wiley & Sons, Inc., Hoboken, New Jersey.
Published simultaneously in Canada..

For general information on our other products and services please contact our Customer Care Department within the U.S. at 877-762-2974, outside the U.S. at 317-572-3993 or fax 317-572-4002.

Wiley also publishes its books in a variety of electronic formats. Some content that appears in print, however, may not be available in electronic format.

Library of Congress Cataloging-in-Publication Data

Pai, G. Shashidhar.
  Handbook of chromosomal syndromes / G. Shashidhar Pai, Raymond C. Lewandowski, Digamber S. Borgaonkar.
     p.   cm.
  Includes bibliographical references and index.
  ISBN 0-471-37217-X (cloth : alk. paper)
  1. Human chromosome abnormalities—Handbooks, manuals, etc.   I. Lewandowski, Raymond C.   II. Borgaonkar, Digamber S.   III. Title.
RB155.5 .P34   2003
616′.042—dc21   2002028847

Printed in the United States of America.

10 9 8 7 6 5 4 3 2 1

To my soul mate, Reese Lovingly, Ray

To my patients and my family who make it all worthwhile.
GSP

Contents

Preface

Over 50 years ago, the chromosomal basis for clinical conditions was established, and in malignancies such as chronic myeloid leukemia it has taken subsequent decades to fully characterize. That discovery has propelled clinical genetic research in a new direction. For example, the number of known chromosomal syndromes almost doubled between 1980 and 1984, also the years in which the third and fourth editions of *Chromosomal Variation in Man* were published. Although that figure reflects a loose count of 48 to 96, the increase is noteworthy in many respects. Multiple congenital anomalies are a universal finding in most autosomal aneuploidies, and can cloud the characterization of individual syndromes. With the introduction and continued development of molecular diagnostic techniques however, it is now possible to collate clinical descriptions of patients with similar chromosomal abnormalities. In the course of preparing the eighth revision of *Chromosomal Variation in Man*, it became evident that the material on chromosomal syndrome descriptions had outgrown its allocated space as an appendix. Out of that realization came the idea for this book.

Soon after the determination of trisomy 21 as a causal defect of Down syndrome, other chromosomal syndromes such as Turner and Klinefelter syndromes were described. Multiple congenital anomalies syndromes of Patau (trisomy 13) and Edwards (trisomy 18) followed. These discoveries established the chromosomal basis of multiple congenital anomalies syndromes. In the subsequent decade only a handful of other syndromes were described: cri-du-chat (5p-), Wolf-Hirschhorn (4p-), DiGeorge (22q-), CML (Ph1), while others such as CLL and Christchurch chromosome (22p-), Sturge-Weber and 1q+, faltered. Part of the reason for this debacle was the lack of a single comprehensive source with data on similar chromosomal anomalies. Attempts were made to start Chromosomal Newsletters but they were not very successful and editors were reluctant to accept case reports for publications. The Chromosomal Variation in Man Online database (www.wiley.com/borgaonkar) is a compilation of citations on chromosomal aneuploidies, coded for easy retrieval. It has been extensively utilized in the development of the present work, and readers are encouraged to update data presented here by their own search of the database.

In the last three decades, several significant developments have taken place. Most noteworthy among these are demands by patients with chromosomal abnormalities and their families for more extensive information from professionals. Chromosomal syndromes have grown in number. Prenatal diagnoses warrant quick delivery of information to enable families to make proper educated decisions on their pregnancies. Decisions about management of newborns with chromosomal syndromes also require up-to-date information on history, longevity, and complexity of problems. It is hoped that this compilation will provide at least a first step for obtaining this information.

G. Shashidhar Pai, M.D.
Raymond C. Lewandowski, Jr., M.D.
Digamber S. Borgaonkar, Ph.D.

Borgaonkar DS, Lacassie YE, Stoll C (1976). Usefulness of chromosome catalog in delineating new syndromes. Birth Defects: Original Article Series XII(5):87–95, The National Foundation-March of Dimes, New York.

Lewandowski RC, Yunis JR, Yunia JJ (1977). Phenotypic mapping in man. In: JJ Yunis, ed. New Chromosomal Syndromes. Academic Press, NY, pp 369–394.

Acknowledgments

I would like to thank my secretaries Cindy Shields, Cristol Duke, and Julia Yong-Goss for secretarial assistance and Dr. Swati Gadewar for contribution to the writing of several chapters. I would also like to thank the patient perseverance and kind editorial guidance and assistance of Ms. Luna Han, Kristin Cooke Fasano, and the entire Wiley team without whom this project would not have been possible.

G. Shashidhar Pai, M.D.

I would like to thank Sara MacKay, Emily Sigler, and Laura Wright for their assistance in completing this book.

Raymond C. Lewandowski, Jr., M.D.

I wish to acknowledge the help of Judith Brightman, Andrea Lynn Dayton, Vinay Hosmani, Deepak Pradhan, and Harshida Shah in the preparation of material for this book, literature search for suitable clinical photographs, and help with citations in my erstwhile Cygtogenetics Laboratory at the Christiana Hospital in Delaware. I also thank the Crystal Trust and the Rieffel Memorial Trust for their financial Support.

Digamber S. Borgaonkar, Ph.D.

HANDBOOK OF CHROMOSOMAL SYNDROMES

CHROMOSOME 1p PARTIAL TRISOMY

Chromosome 1p partial trisomy is a rare chromosomal abnormality with a limited number of patients reported. Although a distinctive phenotype is not apparent, the reported patients do share some frequent features.

MAIN FEATURES: Craniofacial anomalies, growth delay, malformed ears

ABNORMALITIES

Growth: Growth delay

Performance: Developmental delay, motor delay, hypotonicity, mental retardation, seizures

Eyes: Ptosis, hypertelorism, long eyelashes

Craniofacies: Microcephaly, anteverted nares, micrognathia, cleft lip/palate, flat nasal bridge, high-arched palate, malformed ears, epicanthal folds

Other: Syndactyly, thoracic stenosis, adrenal hyperplasia, genital ambiguity, cryptorchidism

CLINICAL COURSE: Early demise has been reported in several patients.

CYTOGENETICS: Inherited rearrangements are unusual.

REFERENCE

Mohammed FM, Farag TI, Gunawardana SS, al-Digashim DD, al-Awadi SA, al-Othman SA, Sundareshan TS. 1989. Direct duplication of chromosome 1, dir dup(1)(p21.2–p32) in a Bedouin with multiple congenital anomalies. *Am. J. Med. Genet.* 32:353–355.

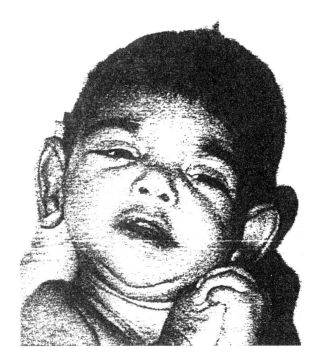

Note microcephaly, sloping forehead, hypertelorism, long eye lashes, anteverted nares, long philtrum, long, malformed pinnae, and micrognathia. (From Mohammed et al., 1989. *Am. J. Med. Genet*. 32:353–355. Copyright © 1989 John Wiley & Sons. Reprinted by permission of Wiley-Liss, Inc.)

CHROMOSOME 1p PARTIAL MONOSOMY

There does not appear to be a single syndrome associated with partial deletion of the short arm of chromosome 1. This may be due in part to the large size of the chromosome. There will most likely end up being several syndromes associated with discrete segments of the chromosome. There are currently an insufficient number of patients with similar deletions to characterize distinctive syndromes.

MAIN FEATURES: Mental retardation, developmental delay, low-set, malformed ears, long face

ABNORMALITIES

Growth: Short stature

Performance: Psychomotor and mental retardation, developmental delay, mild hypotonia

Craniofacies: Dysmorphic facial features, abnormal nasal bridge, long face, large fontanelle, abnormal palpebral fissures, low-set malformed ears

Limbs: Bilateral simian creases, clinodactyly of the fifth finger, abnormally flexed fingers and toes

Other: Seizures and cardiac defects

OCCASIONAL ABNORMALITIES: Apnea, frontal bossing, hydrocephalus, prominent nasal tip, hearing loss, high palate, micrognathia, microstomia, wide-spaced nipples

CLINICAL COURSE: Death in infancy has been documented.

CYTOGENETICS: Most of the deletions are de novo.

REFERENCES

Barton JS, O'Loughlin J, Howell RT, L'e Orme R. 1995. Developmental delay and dysmorphic features associated with a previously undescribed deletion on chromosome 1. *J. Med. Genet.* 32:636–637.

Dockery H, Van der Westhuyzen J. 1991. Monosomy of 1p13.3–22.3 in twins. *Clin. Genet.* 39:223–227.

Keppler-Noreuil KM, Carroll AJ, Finley WH, Rutledge SL. 1995. Chromosome 1p terminal deletion: report of new findings and confirmation of two characteristic phenotypes. *J. Med. Genet.* 32:619–622.

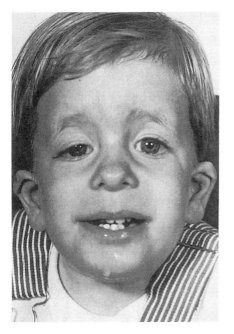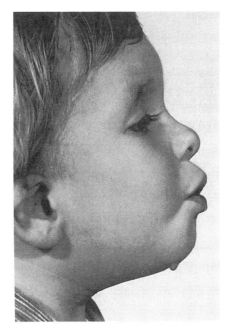

Patient's facial features at 1 year and 2 months, demonstrating right ptosis, deep-set eyes, arched eyebrows, long eyelashes, low-set ears with overlapping helices, and micrognathia. (From Mattia et al., 1992. *Am. J. Med. Genet.* 44:551–554. Copyright © 1992 John Wiley & Sons, Inc. Reprinted by permission of Wiley-Liss, Inc.)

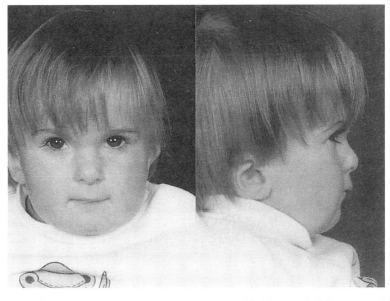

Note the cherubic features, low-set ears, prominent nasal bridge and philtrum, and long eyelashes. (From Barton et al., 1995. *J. Med. Genet.* 32:636–637. Copyright © 1995 John Wiley & Sons, Inc. Reprinted by permission of Wiley-Liss, Inc.)

Lai MM, Robards MF, Berry AC, Fear CN, Hart C. 1991. Two cases of interstitial deletion 1p. *J. Med. Genet.* 28:128–130.

Mattia FR, Wardinsky TD, Tuttle DJ, Grix A Jr, Smith KA, Walling P. 1992. Interstitial deletion of the short arm of chromosome 1 (46XY, del(1)(p13p22.3)). *Am. J. Med. Genet.* 44:551–554.

Tabata H, Sone K, Kobayashi T, Yanagisawa T, Tamura T, Shimizu N, Kanbe Y, Tashiro M, Ono S, Kuroume T. 1991. Short arm deletion of chromosome 1: del(1)(p13.3p22.3) in a female infant with an extreme tetralogy of Fallot. *Clin. Genet.* 39:132–135.

CHROMOSOME 1q PARTIAL TRISOMY

Patients with partial trisomy for the distal end of chromosome 1, q41 → qter, appear to have a distinctive phenotype. Most patients with this defect result from a parental chromosomal rearrangement and, as a result, their phenotypes are not "pure."

MAIN FEATURES: Prominent forehead, large fontanelle, low-set ears

ABNORMALITIES

Performance: Developmental delay and mental retardation

Craniofacies: Low-set, malformed ears, abnormal nose, micrognathia, macrocephaly, long philtrum, brachycephaly, carplike mouth, frontal bossing

Genitourinary: Genitourinary abnormalities, cryptorchidism

Limbs: Abnormal fingers and toes, dysplastic nails, simian creases

Other: Cardiac defects, heart murmur, cerebellar hypoplasia, hydrocephalus, high palate

OCCASIONAL ABNORMALITIES: Hypertelorism, growth retardation, facial capillary hemangiomas

CLINICAL COURSE: Death in early infancy is not unusual. Survival into adult life has also been reported.

CYTOGENETICS: Most patients result from parental chromosomal rearrangements.

REFERENCES

Chen H, Kusyk CJ, Tuck-Muller CM, Martinez JE, Dorand RD, Wertelecki W. 1994. Confirmation of proximal 1q duplication using fluorescence in situ hybridization. *Am. J. Med. Genet.* 50:28–31.

Johnson VP. 1991. Duplication of the distal part of the long arm of chromosome 1. *Am. J. Med. Genet.* 39:258–269.

Kennerknecht I, Barbi G, Rodens K. 1993. Dup(1q)(q42 → qter) syndrome: case report and review of literature. *Am. J. Med. Genet.* 47:1157–1160.

Rasmussen SA, Frias JL, Lafer CZ, Eunpu DL, Zackai EH. 1990. Partial duplication 1q: report of four patients and review of the literature. *Am. J. Med. Genet.* 36:137–143.

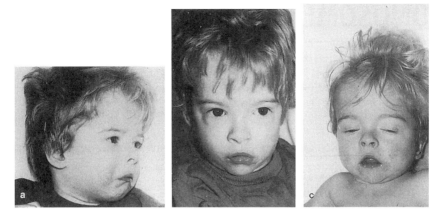

Patient at 1 year and 4 months (a,c) and at 4 years and 4 months (b). Note triangular face, frontal bossing, telecanthus, upturned nose, micrognathia, and small mouth with downturned corners. (From Kennerknecht et al., 1993. *Am. J. Med. Genet.* 47:1157–1160. Copyright © 1993 John Wiley & Sons, Inc. Reprinted by permission of Wiley-Liss, Inc.)

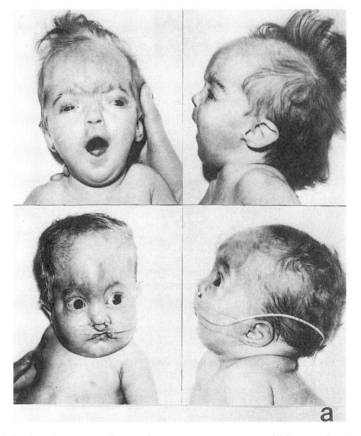

Note prominent forehead, depressed temples, prominent eyes, mild hypertelorism, short nose, anteverted nares, and cupped ears. (From Johnson, 1991. *Am. J. Med. Genet.* 39:258–269. Copyright © 1991 John Wiley & Sons, Inc. Reprinted by permission of Wiley-Liss, Inc.)

CHROMOSOME 1q PARTIAL MONOSOMY

Deletion of a portion of the long arm of chromosome 1 involving bands q42 → qter appears to produce a distinct syndrome.

MAIN FEATURES: Growth and psychomotor retardation, short neck, micrognathia

ABNORMALITIES

Growth: Intrauterine growth retardation (IUGR), postnatal growth retardation, microcephaly

Performance: Moderate to severe psychomotor retardation, seizures, hearing loss

Craniofacies: Brachycephaly, short, broad nose, upward-slanting palpebral fissures, epicanthal folds, telecanthus, carp-shaped mouth with downturned corners, cleft palate, micrognathia, abnormal ears, short neck

Other: Genital abnormalities, abnormal hands and feet, high-pitched cry in infancy, central nervous system abnormalities seen on CT scan or MRI, hypotonia, vertebrae abnormalities, autonomic dysfunction

CLINICAL COURSE: These patients do not usually die early and survival into teenage years is reported.

CYTOGENETICS: Most defects are de novo.

REFERENCES

Halal F, Vekemans M, Kaplan P, Zeesman S. 1990. Distal deletion of chromosome 1q in an adult. *Am. J. Med. Genet.* 35:379–382.

Ioan DM, Maximilian C, Kleczkowska A, Fryns JP. 1992. Distal deletion of the long arm of chromosome number 1(q43 → qter) associated with severe mental retardation and a nonspecific dysmorphic syndrome. *Ann. Genet.* 35:167–169.

Leichtman LG, Strum D, Brothman AR. 1993. Multiple craniofacial anomalies associated with an interstitial deletion of chromosome 1(q21 → q25). *Am. J. Med. Genet.* 45:677–678.

Murayama K, Greenwood RS, Rao KW, Aylsworth AS. 1991. Neurological aspects of del(1q) syndrome. *Am. J. Med. Genet.* 40:488–492.

Rotmensch S, Liberati M, Luo JS, Tallini G, Mahoney MJ, Hobbins JC. 1991. Prenatal diagnosis of a fetus with terminal deletion of chromosome 1(q41). *Prenat. Diagn.* 11:867–873.

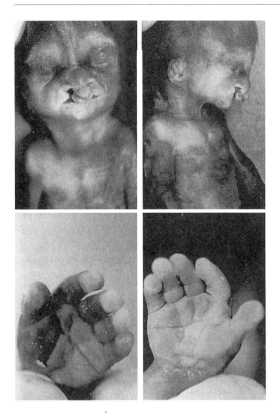

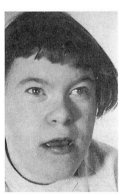
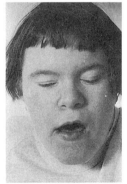

Note brachycephaly, prominent metopic suture ridge, bilateral cleft lip, low-set, malformed ears, micrognathia, simian crease, and prominent fingertip pad. (From Leichtman et al., 1993. *Am. J. Med. Genet.* 45:677–678. Copyright © 1993 John Wiley & Sons, Inc. Reprinted by permission of Wiley-Liss, Inc.)

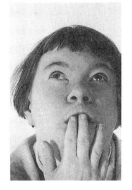
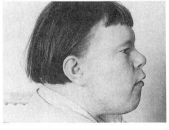

Note Down syndrome-like appearance, coarse face, upward-slanting palpebral fissures, epicanthal folds, strabismus, short nose, full cheeks, and short neck. (From Halal et al., 1990. *Am. J. Med. Genet.* 35:379–382. Copyright © 1990 John Wiley & Sons, Inc. Reprinted by permission of Wiley-Liss, Inc.)

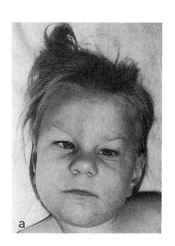 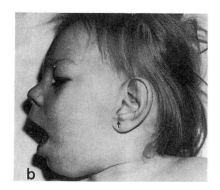

Facial appearance of patient (a: front view, b: side view). Microcephaly, full-round face (especially in lower part), unruly hair, periorbital fullness especially of the upper eyelids, infraorbital folds, relatively large ears, with prominent antihelix, oblique upward-slanting palpebral fissures, prominent broad nasal bridge with anteverted nasal tip, hypoplastic philtrum, down-curved thin vermillion border of upper lip, slight micrognathia, short neck, and increased submandibular fat. (From Murayama et al., 1991. *Am. J. Med. Genet.* 40:488–492. Copyright © 1991 John Wiley & Sons, Inc. Reprinted by permission of Wiley-Liss, Inc.)

RING CHROMOSOME 1

Ring chromosome 1 is a rare abnormality. Due partly to the variable size of the resulting chromosome, there is not a distinctive phenotype associated with this defect.

MAIN FEATURES: Developmental delay, growth retardation, microcephaly, dwarfism, clinodactyly

ABNORMALITIES

Growth: Growth retardation

Performance: Developmental delay, microcephaly, hypotonia

Eyes: Megacornea, cataracts, glaucoma

Craniofacies: Asymmetry of the skull, ear malformations, upward-slanting palpebral fissures, abnormal philtrum

Other: Dwarfism, clinodactyly, flexion contractures

CLINICAL COURSE: Severe hypotonia with motor delay and dwarfism

CYTOGENETICS: All patients arose de novo

REFERENCES

Chen H, Tuck-Muller CM, Batista DA, Wertelecki W. 1995. Identification of supernumerary ring chromosome 1 mosaicism using fluorescence in situ hybridization. *Am. J. Med. Genet.* 56:219–233.

Gordon RR, Cooke P. 1964. Ring 1 chromosome and microcephalic dwarfism. *Lancet.* ii:1212–1213.

Kjessler B, Gustavson KH, Wigertz A. 1978. Apparently non-deleted ring-1 chromosome and extreme growth failure in a mentally retarded girl. *Clin. Genet.* 14:8–15.

Wolf CB, Peterson JA, LoGrippo GA, Weiss L. 1967. Ring 1 chromosome and dwarfism—a possible syndrome. *J. Pediatr.* 71:719–722.

CHROMOSOME 2p PARTIAL TRISOMY

Most reported cases involve patients with duplication for p21 → pter. Because of the large size of this chromosomal segment, there will undoubtedly be several distinct syndromes eventually identified. There is, nevertheless, a sufficiently characteristic phenotype to assign to patients with the above segment involved.

MAIN FEATURES: Flat nasal bridge, hypertelorism, ear malformations, genital malformations

ABNORMALITIES

Growth: Growth retardation

Performance: Psychomotor retardation

Eyes: Hypertelorism

Craniofacies: Microcephaly, epicanthic folds, micrognathia, ear malformations, nose abnormalities, flat nasal bridge, abnormal philtrum

Other: Long hyperreflexive fingers, visceral malformations, genital malformations, hypotonia

OCCASIONAL ABNORMALITIES: Neural tube defects, bronchopulmonary aplasia/ hypoplasia, diaphragmatic hernia, "situs" and looping congenital heart defects, neuroblastoma

CLINICAL COURSE: Death often occurs in early infancy, but survival into adult life is reported.

CYTOGENETICS: Most patients result from a parental chromosomal rearrangement.

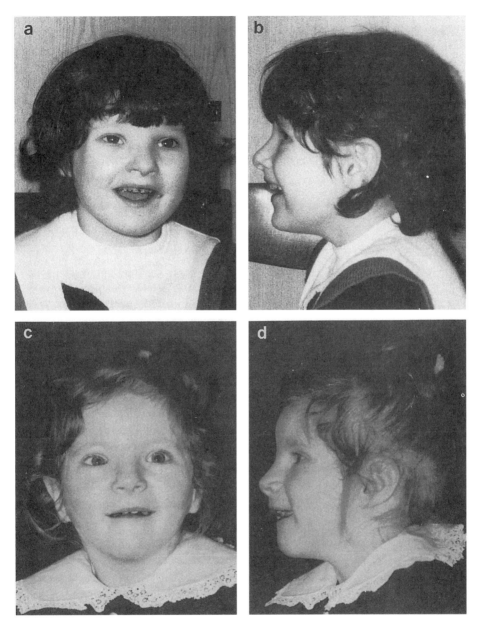

Patient 1 is 4 years old (a,b). Note brachycephaly, low hair growth, and prognathia. Patient 2 is 2 years and 6 months old (c,d). Note asymmetric face, sloping forehead, upward-slanting palpebral fissures, left convergent squint, sharp, narrow nose, short, distinct philtrum, and small, pointed chin. (From Lurie et al., 1995. *Am. J. Med. Genet.* 55:229–236. Copyright © 1995 John Wiley & Sons, Inc. Reprinted by permission of Wiley-Liss, Inc.)

REFERENCES

Chen CP, Liu FF, Jan SW, Lin SP, Lan CC. 1996. Prenatal diagnosis of partial monosomy 3p and partial trisomy 2p in a fetus associated with shortening of the long bones and a single umbilical artery. *Prenat. Diagn.* 16:270–275.

Fineman RM, Buyse M, Morgan M. 1983. Variable phenotype associated with duplication of different regions of 2p. *Am. J. Med. Genet.* 15:451–456.

Lurie IW, Ilyina HG, Gurevich DB, Rumyantseva NV, Naumchik IV, Castellan C, Hoeller A, Schinzel A. 1995. Trisomy 2p: analysis of unusual phenotypic findings. *Am. J. Med. Genet.* 55:229–236.

Parruti G, Di Ilio C, Calabrese G, Stuppia L, Guanciali Franchi P, Aceto A, Palka G. 1989. A new case of partial 2p trisomy due to de novo interstitial duplication 2p21–22. *Ann. Genet.* 32:55–58.

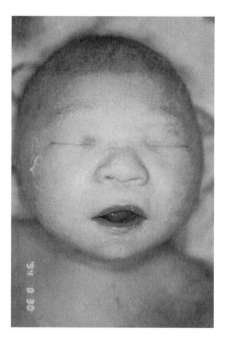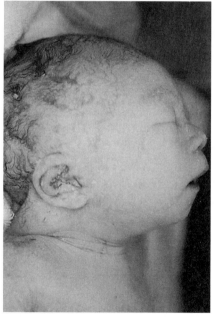

Note micrognathia, blepharoptosis, epicanthal folds, hypertelorism, downturned mouth, deformed, low-set ears with periauricular pits, and a prominent nose. (From Chen et al., 1996. *Prenat. Diagn.* 16:270–275. Copyright © 1996 John Wiley and Sons Limited. Reproduced with permission.)

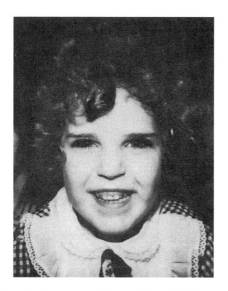

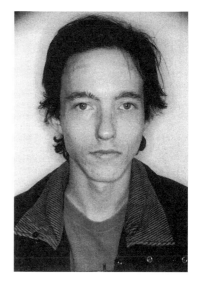

Patient is 4 years and 6 months old. Note squint. (From Fineman et al., 1983. *Am. J. Med. Genet.* 15:451–456. Copyright © 1983 John Wiley & Sons, Inc. Reprinted by permission of Wiley-Liss, Inc.)

Note synophrys, narrow nasal root, and broad nasal tip. (From Sawyer et al., 1994. *Am. J. Med. Genet.* 49:422–427. Copyright © 1994 John Wiley & Sons, Inc. Reprinted by permission of Wiley-Liss, Inc.)

CHROMOSOME 2p PARTIAL MONOSOMY

Two groups of patients are reported with partial deletion 2p. One group involves a distal deletion and the other an interstitial deletion.

MAIN FEATURES: Developmental delay, mental retardation, rectangular-appearing face

ABNORMALITIES

Growth: Growth retardation

Performance: Developmental delay, mental retardation

Craniofacies: Rectangular facies, ear malformations, abnormal palpebral fissures, abnormal nasal bridge

Other: Abnormal fingers and toes, reduced visual acuity

CLINICAL COURSE: Adults are reported.

CYTOGENETICS: Familial chromosomal translocations have been reported.

REFERENCES

Francis GL, Flannery DB, Byrd JR, Fisher ST. 1990. An apparent de novo terminal deletion of chromosome 2 (pter–p24:). *J. Med. Genet.* 27:137–138.

Los FJ, Van Hemel JO, Jacobs HJ, Drop SL, van Dongen JJ. 1994. De novo deletion (2)(p11.2p13): clinical, cytogenetic, and immunological data. *J. Med. Genet.* 31:72–73.

Prasher VP, Krishnan VH, Clarke DJ, Maliszewska CT, Corbett JA. 1993. Deletion of chromosome 2(p11–p13): case report and review. *J. Med. Genet.* 30:604–606.

Saal HM, King LJ, Zimmerman D, Johnson RC, Carr AG, Samango-Sprouse CA, Stanley W. 1996. Loss of the N-myc oncogene in a patient with a small interstitial deletion of the short arm of chromosome 2. *Am. J. Med. Genet.* 66:373–377.

Sawyer JR, Jones E, Hawks FF, Quirk JG Jr, Cunniff C. 1994. Duplication and deletion of chromosome band 2(p21p22) resulting from a familial interstitial insertion (2;11)(p21;p15). *Am. J. Med. Genet.* 49:422–427.

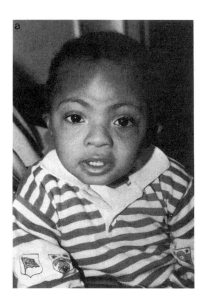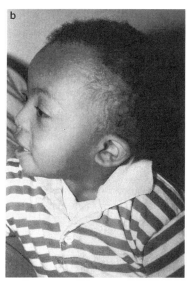

Note microbrachycephaly, mild synophrys, arching of the eyebrows, rectangular face, and low-set ears and eyes. (From Saal et al., 1996. *Am. J. Med. Genet.* 66:373–377. Copyright © 1996 John Wiley & Sons, Inc. Reprinted by permission of Wiley-Liss, Inc.)

CHROMOSOME 2q PARTIAL TRISOMY

Partial trisomy for 2q is a rare finding, although it results in some predictable features. In most patients this defect is de novo.

MAIN FEATURES: Epicanthal folds, clinodactyly of the fifth finger, abnormal fingers and toes, developmental delay

ABNORMALITIES

Growth: Growth retardation

Performance: Developmental delay, mental retardation

Craniofacies: Broad and flat nasal bridge, low-set ears, hypertelorism, epicanthal folds, long philtrum, micrognathia, thin upper lip

Limbs: Abnormal fingers and toes, clinodacyly of the fifth finger

Other: Cardiac defects, scoliosis

OCCASIONAL ABNORMALITIES: Ptosis, external genital anomalies

CLINICAL COURSE: Death in early infancy is not unusual, but survival into adult life has been reported.

CYTOGENETICS: In most instances, the patient represents a de novo defect, although parental chromosomal rearrangements do occur.

REFERENCES

Cooke LB, Richards H, Lunt PW, Burvill-Holmes L, Howell RT, McDermott A. 1995. Duplication 2(q11.2–q21): a previously unreported abnormality. *J. Med. Genet.* 32:825–826.

Dahl N, Eliasson IL, Gustavson KH. 1988. A case of complete trisomy 2p/triploidy mosaicism. *Acta. Paediatr. Scand.* 77:925–929.

Dahoun-Hadorn S, Bretton-Chappuis B. 1992. De novo inversion-duplication of 2q35-2qter without growth retardation. *Ann. Genet.* 35:55–57.

Ramer JC, Mowrey PN, Robins DB, Ligato S, Towfighi J, Ladda R. 1990. Five children with del(2)(q31q33) and one individual with dup(2)(q31q33) from a single family: review of brain, cardiac, and limb malformations. *Am. J. Med. Genet.* 37:392–400.

Romain DR, Mackenzie NG, Moss D, Columbano-Green LM, Smythe RH, Parfitt RG, Dixon JW. 1994. Partial trisomy for 2q in a patient with dir dup(2)(q33.1q35). *J. Med. Genet.* 31:652–653.

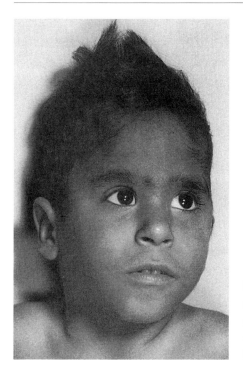

Patient at 2 years and 3 months. Note hirsutism, synophrys, and mild micrognathia. (From Ramer et al., 1990. *Am. J. Med. Genet.* 37:392–400. Copyright © 1990 John Wiley & Sons, Inc. Reprinted by permission of Wiley-Liss, Inc.)

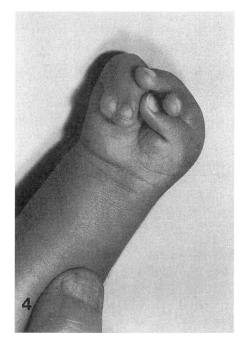

Note right hand of patient showing fusion of the first and second and third and fourth fingers as well as the fixed position of the thumb. (From Ramer et al., 1990. *Am. J. Med. Genet.* 37:392–400. Copyright © 1990 John Wiley & Sons, Inc. Reprinted by permission of Wiley-Liss, Inc.)

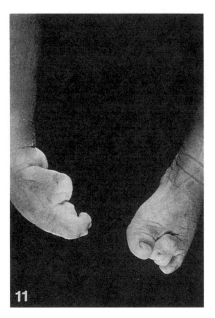

Note absent right hallux, centralized syndactylic right toes, and fusion of the middle two toes on the left foot. (From Ramer et al., 1990. *Am. J. Med. Genet.* 37:392–400. Copyright © 1990 John Wiley & Sons, Inc. Reprinted by permission of Wiley-Liss, Inc.)

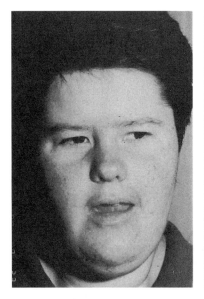
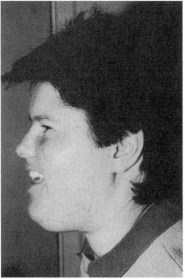

Note epicanthal folds, depressed nasal bridge, thin upper lip with cupid's bow, long philtrum, and short neck. (From Romain et al., 1994. *J. Med. Genet.* 31:652–653. Reprinted with permission of BMJ Publishing Group.)

CHROMOSOME 2q PARTIAL MONOSOMY

Chromosome 2q is a large chromosomal segment and a number of interstitial deletions as well as terminal deletions have been reported. Not unexpectedly, there is not a common phenotype for all these patients. Furthermore, there is not a distinctive phenotype for any of the related deletions other than the terminal deletion q24 → qter.

MAIN FEATURES: Mental retardation, seizures, hypotonia, frontal bossing, ear malformations

ABNORMALITIES IN del(q24 → qter)

Growth: Postnatal growth retardation

Performance: Mental retardation, repetitive behavior

Craniofacies: Frontal bossing, microcephaly, macrocephaly, downward-slanting palpebral fissures, long eyelashes, micrognathia

Other: Cardiac defects

ABNORMALITIES IN OTHER DELETIONS

Growth: Postnatal growth retardation

Performance: Mental retardation, developmental delay, seizures, hypotonia, psychomotor retardation

Eyes: Hypertelorism

Craniofacies: Unusual facies, ear and nose malformations, abnormal palpebral fissures, depressed nasal bridge, high-arched palate, micrognathia

Other: Deviation and syndactyly of digits, abnormal nipples

CLINICAL COURSE: Survival is variable, depending on the size and location of the deletion. Survival into late childhood is reported.

CYTOGENETICS: In almost all cases the defects are de novo.

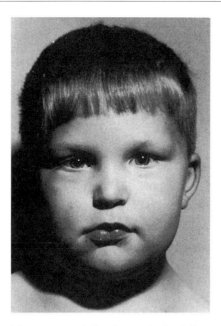

Patient at 6 years. Note round face, upward-slanting palpebral fissures, unilateral esotropia, short nose, and depressed nasal bridge. (From Phelan et al., 1995. *Am. J. Med. Genet.* 58:1–7. Copyright © 1995 John Wiley & Sons, Inc. Reprinted by permission of Wiley-Liss, Inc.)

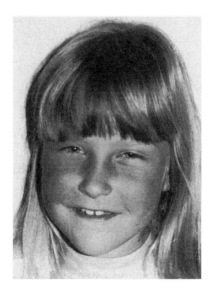

Patient at 6 years and 6 months. Note mild facial asymmetry, mild bilateral ptosis, and excessive folding of the helices. (From Phelan et al., 1995. *Am. J. Med. Genet.* 58:1–7. Copyright © 1995 John Wiley & Sons, Inc. Reprinted by permission of Wiley-Liss, Inc.)

REFERENCES

Boles RG, Pober BR, Gibson LH, Willis CR, McGrath J, Roberts DJ, Yang-Feng TL. 1995. Deletion of chromosome 2q24–q31 causes characteristic digital anomalies: case report and review. *Am. J. Med. Genet.* 55:155–160.

Conrad B, Dewald G, Christensen E, Lopez M, Higgins J, Pierpont ME. 1995. Clinical phenotype associated with terminal 2q37 deletion. *Clin. Genet.* 48:134–139.

Fisher AM, Ellis KH, Browne CE, Barber JC, Barker M, Kennedy CR, Foley H, Patton MA. 1994. Small terminal deletions of the long arm of chromosome 2: two new cases. *Am. J. Med. Genet.* 53:366–369.

Kirkpatrick SJ, Kent CM, Laxova R, Sekhon GS. 1992. Waardenburg syndrome type I in a child with deletion (2)(q35q36.2). *Am. J. Med. Genet.* 44:699–700.

Melnyk AR, Muraskas J. 1993. Interstitial deletion of chromosome 2 region in a malformed infant. *Am. J. Med. Genet.* 45:49–51.

Phelan MC, Rogers RC, Clarkson KB, Bowyer FP, Levine MA, Estabrooks LL, Severson MC, Dobyns WB. 1995. Albright hereditary osteodystrophy and del(2)(q37.3) in four unrelated individuals. *Am. J. Med. Genet.* 58:1–7.

Wamsler C, Muller B, Freyberger G, Schmid M. 1991. Interstitial deletion del(2)(q24q31) with a phenotype similar to del(2)(q31q33). *Am. J. Med. Genet.* 39:204–206.

Waters BL, Allen EF, Gibson PC, Johnston T. 1993. Autopsy findings in a severely affected infant with a 2q terminal deletion. *Am. J. Med. Genet.* 47:1099–1103.

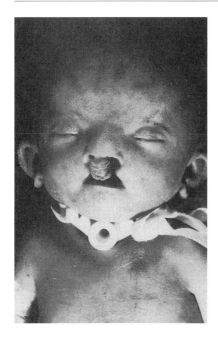

Patient at birth. Note macrocephaly, hypertelorism, short palpebral fissures, microphthalmia, bilateral cleft lip and palate, micrognathia, and low-set, posteriorly angulated ears. (From Waters et al., 1993. *Am. J. Med. Genet.* 47:1099–1103. Copyright © 1993 John Wiley & Sons, Inc. Reprinted by permission of Wiley-Liss, Inc.)

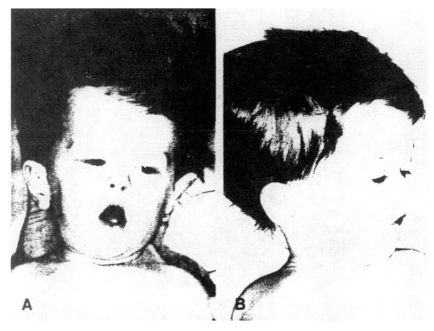

A   B

Note frontal bossing, triangular-shaped skull, profuse scalp hair, depressed nasal bridge, upturned nose, bilateral epicanthal folds, short palpebral fissures, low-set ears, downturned mouth, and redundant nuchal skin folds. (From Conrad et al., 1995. *Clin. Genet.* 48:134–139. Copyright © 1995 Munksgaard International Publishers Ltd., Copenhagen, Denmark, with permission.)

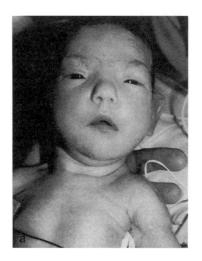

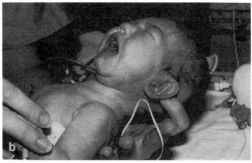

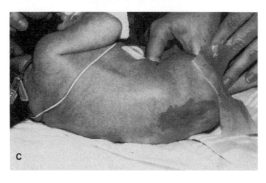

Patient at age 1 week. Note hypertelorism, round face, arched eyebrows, wide nasal tip, upturned nares, long philtrum, small mouth with downturned corners (a), mildly dysplastic ears (b), and repaired lumbosacral meningomyelocele (c). (From Melnyk and Muraskas, 1993. *Am. J. Med. Genet.* 45:49–51. Copyright © 1993 John Wiley & Sons, Inc. Reprinted by permission of Wiley-Liss, Inc.)

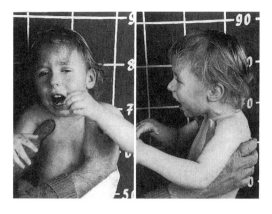

Patient at age 3 years and 3 months. Note low-set, abnormal ears, narrow palpebral fissures, with anti-mongoloid slant, hypotelorism, ptosis, large, beaked nose, receding chin, and receding forehead. (From Wamsler et al., 1991. *Am. J. Med. Genet.* 39:204–206. Copyright © 1991 John Wiley & Sons, Inc. Reprinted by permission of Wiley-Liss, Inc.)

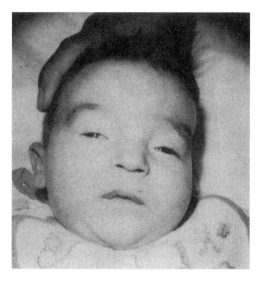

Note short and downward-slanting palpebral fissures. (From Boles et al., 1995. *Am. J. Med. Genet.* 55:155–160. Copyright © 1995 John Wiley & Sons, Inc. Reprinted by permission of Wiley-Liss, Inc.)

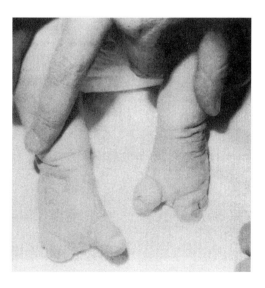

Note split foot with a wide gap between broad halluces and brachysyndactylous digits 3–5. The second digits are absent. (From Boles et al., 1995. *Am. J. Med. Genet.* 55:155–160. Copyright © 1995 John Wiley & Sons, Inc. Reprinted by permission of Wiley-Liss, Inc.)

RING CHROMOSOME 2

Patients with ring chromosome 2 are extremely rare. Among the few documented cases, there appears to be phenotypic similarity, including growth retardation and microcephaly.

MAIN FEATURES: Microcephaly, growth retardation, and facial dysmorphism

ABNORMALITIES

Growth: Intrauterine growth retardation (IUGR), growth retardation

Performance: Failure to thrive, poor feeding, developmental delay, mental retardation

Craniofacies: Microcephaly, flat occiput, short neck, abnormal, low-set ears, flat nasal bridge, epicanthal folds, abnormal philtrum, micrognathia

Genitourinary: Hypoplasia of labia minora, undescended testes

Limbs: Rocker-bottom feet, clinodactyly of the fifth finger

OCCASIONAL ABNORMALITIES: Heart defects, abnormalities of the palate

CLINICAL COURSE: Death in early infancy has been documented.

CYTOGENETICS: In most instances, the patient represents a de novo defect, although parental chromosomal rearrangements and mosaicism do occur.

REFERENCES

Cote GB, Katsantoni A, Deligeorgis D. 1981. The cytogenetic and clinical implications of a ring chromosome 2. *Ann. Genet.* 24:231–235.

Jansen M, Beemer FA, van der Heiden C, Van Hemel JO, Van den Brande JL. 1982. Ring chromosome 2: clinical, chromosomal, and biochemical aspects. *Hum. Genet.* 60:91–95.

Maraschio P, Danesino C, Garau A, Saputo V, Vigi V, Volpato S. 1979. Three cases of ring chromosome 2, one derived from a paternal 2/6 translocation. *Hum. Genet.* 48:157–167.

Vigfusson NV, Kapstafer KJ, Lloyd MA. 1980. Ring chromosome 2 in a child with growth failure and few congenital abnormalities. *Am. J. Med. Genet.* 7:383–389.

Wyandt HE, Kasprzak R, Lamb A, Willson K, Wilson WG, Kelly TE. 1982. Human chromosome 2 rod/ring mosaicism: probable origin by prezygotic breakage and intrachromosomal exchange. *Cancer Genet. Cytogenet.* 33:222–231.

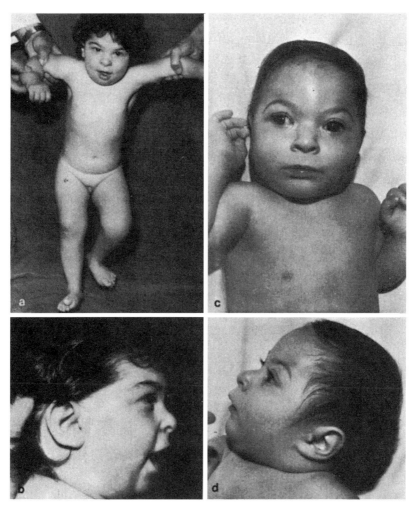

Note microcephaly, bulging metopic suture, flat nasal bridge, short philtrum, low-set ears, epicanthal folds, upward-slanting palpebral fissures, micrognathia, short neck, and widely spaced nipples (a,b). Note microcephaly, bulging metopic suture, large, low-set ears, bilateral epicanthal folds, upward-slanting palpebral fissures, arched eyebrows, exotropia, flat nasal bridge, long philtrum, micrognathia, short neck, and widely spaced nipples (c,d). (From Maraschio et al., 1979. *Hum. Genet.* 48:157–167. Copyright © 1979 Springer-Verlag. Reprinted with permission.)

CHROMOSOME 3p PARTIAL TRISOMY

Duplication of chromosome 3p is relatively rare and there does not appear to be a single associated syndrome. More patients will be required in order to characterize a distinct syndrome.

MAIN FEATURES: Facial dysmorphism, low posterior hairline, hypotonia

ABNORMALITIES

Performance: Developmental delay, hypotonia

Craniofacies: Abnormal head shape, short neck, abnormal, low-set ears, hypertelorism, small mouth, square face with full cheeks

Other: Low posterior hairline, widely spaced nipples

Limbs: Simian creases, abnormal fingers and toes

OCCASIONAL ABNORMALITIES: Holoprosencephaly, cyclopia, epicanthal folds

CLINICAL COURSE: Death in early infancy has been documented.

CYTOGENETICS: In most instances, the patient represents a de novo defect although parental chromosomal rearrangements do occur.

REFERENCES

Game K, Friedman JM, Kalousek DK. 1990. Mild phenotypic abnormalities in combined del 9p2 and dup 3p2. *Am. J. Med. Genet.* 35:370–372.

Gillerot Y, Hustin J, Koulischer L, Viteux V. 1987. Prenatal diagnosis of a dup(3p) with holoprosencephaly. *Am. J. Med. Genet.* 26:225–227.

Kurtzman DN, Van Dyke DL, Rich CA, Weiss L. 1987. Duplication 3p21–3pter and cyclopia. *Am. J. Med. Genet.* 27:33–37.

Scarbrough PR, Carroll AJ, Finley WH, Bridges DR. 1987. A de novo 3p;8p unbalanced translocation resulting in partial dup(3p) and partial del(8p). *J. Med. Genet.* 24:174–177.

Watson MS, Dowton SB, Rohrbaugh J. 1990. Case of direct insertion within a chromosome 3 leading to a chromosome 3p duplication in an offspring. *Am. J. Med. Genet.* 36:172–174.

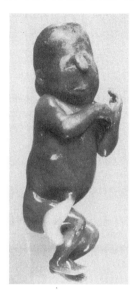

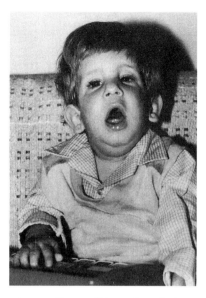

Affected fetus at 19 weeks gestation. Note absent nose and frontal proboscis. (From Gillerot et al., 1987. *Am. J. Med. Genet.* 26:225–227. Copyright © 1987 John Wiley & Sons, Inc. Reprinted by permission of Wiley-Liss, Inc.)

Patient at 1 year. Note mild ptosis, relative hypertelorism, low-set ears with abnormal helices, and cupid bow shape to the downturned upper lip. (From Watson et al., 1990. *Am. J. Med. Genet.* 36:172–174. Copyright © 1990 John Wiley & Sons, Inc. Reprinted by permission of Wiley-Liss, Inc.)

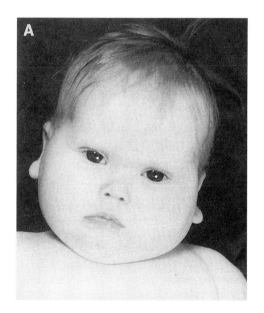

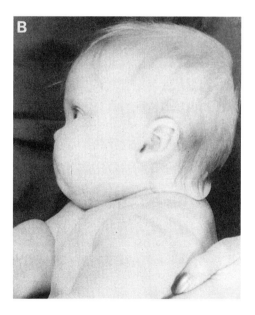

Patient at 4.5 months. Note narrow bifrontal diameter, high forehead, occipital flattening, wide-spaced eyes, unusual auricles, small mouth, small mandible, and full cheeks. (From Game et al., 1990. *Am. J. Med. Genet.* 35:370–372. Copyright © 1990 John Wiley & Sons, Inc. Reprinted by permission of Wiley-Liss, Inc.)

CHROMOSOME 3p PARTIAL MONOSOMY

Patients with a deletion containing 3p25.3 appear to have a distinct phenotype. Most of these deletions are de novo.

MAIN FEATURES: Long philtrum, micrognathia, abnormal palpebral fissures

ABNORMALITIES

Growth: Growth retardation

Performance: Psychomotor retardation, mental retardation, hypotonia, poor feeding

Craniofacies: Microcephaly, ptosis, low-set ears, blepharophimosis, abnormal palpebral fissures, hypertelorism, long philtrum, micrognathia, flat nasal bridge

Other: Hearing loss

OCCASIONAL ABNORMALITIES: Flat occiput, simian creases, and abnormal fingers and toes, mandibulofacial dysostosis in one case

CLINICAL COURSE: Death in infancy has been noted.

CYTOGENETICS: In almost all cases the defects are de novo.

REFERENCES

Arn PH, Mankinen C, Jabs EW. 1993. Mild mandibulofacial dysostosis in a child with a deletion of 3p. *Am. J. Med. Genet.* 46:534–536.

Barrios L, Miro R, Caballin MR, Vayreda J, Subias A, Egozcue J. 1986. Constitutional del(3)(p14–p21) in a patient with bladder carcinoma. *Cancer Genet. Cytogenet.* 21:171–173.

Moncla A, Philip N, Mattei JF. 1995. Blepharophimosis-mental retardation syndrome and terminal deletion of chromosome 3p. *J. Med. Genet.* 32:245–246.

Mowrey PN, Chorney MJ, Venditti CP, Latif F, Modi WS, Lerman MI, Zbar B, Robins DB, Rogan PK, Ladda RL. 1993. Clinical and molecular analyses of deletion 3p25-pter syndrome. *Am. J. Med. Genet.* 46:623–629.

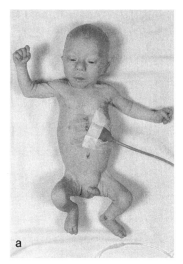 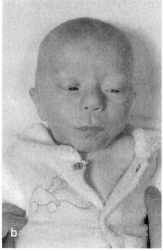 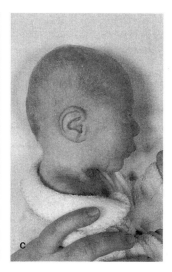

Patient at 2 months. Note flat nasal bridge, bilateral ptosis, apparent hypertelorism, small ears with simple folded helix, long philtrum, thin upper lip, "carp-like" mouth, and micrognathia. (From Mowrey et al., 1993. *Am. J. Med. Genet.* 46:623–629. Copyright © 1993 John Wiley & Sons, Inc. Reprinted by permission of Wiley-Liss, Inc.)

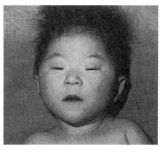 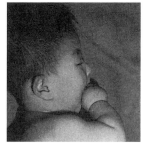

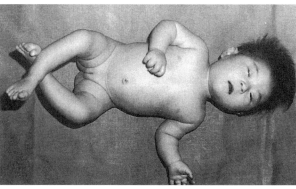

Patient at 10 months. Note flat occiput, triangular face, narrow forehead, low anterior hairline, hypertelorism, bilateral blepharoptosis, short palpebral fissures, malformed ears, broad, flat nose, long philtrum, downturned mouth, and small pointed chin. (From Narahara et al., 1990. *Am. J. Med. Genet.* 35:269–273. Copyright © 1990 John Wiley & Sons, Inc. Reprinted by permission of Wiley-Liss, Inc.)

Narahara K, Kikkawa K, Murakami M, Hiramoto K, Namba H, Tsuji K, Yokoyama Y, Kimoto H. 1990. Loss of the 3p25.3 band is critical in the manifestation of del(3p) syndrome: karyotype-phenotype correlation in cases with deficiency of the distal portion of the short arm of chromosome 3. *Am. J. Med. Genet.* 35:269–273.

Neri G, Reynolds JF, Westphal J, Hinz J, Daniel A. 1984. Interstitial deletion of chromosome 3p: report of a patient and delineation of a proximal 3p deletion syndrome. *Am. J. Med. Genet.* 19:189–193.

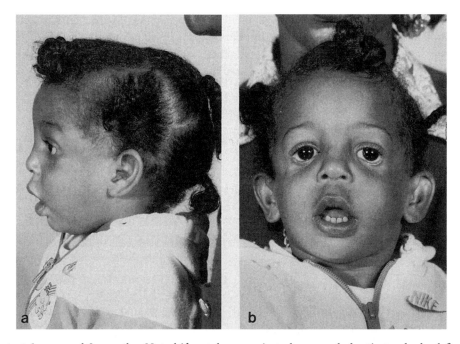

Patient at 1 year and 9 months. Note bifrontal narrowing, downward-slanting palpebral fissures, shallow orbits with prominent globes, sparse lower lashes, malar hypoplasia, and micrognathia. (From Arn et al., 1993. *Am. J. Med. Genet.* 46:534–536. Copyright © 1993 John Wiley & Sons, Inc. Reprinted by permission of Wiley-Liss, Inc.)

CHROMOSOME 3q PARTIAL TRISOMY

The features of partial duplication 3q overlap those of Brachmann-de Lange syndrome. Convulsions, eye, palate, and cardiac malformations are more common in duplication 3q and limb defects, hirsutism and synophrys are more common in Brachmann-de Lange syndrome.

MAIN FEATURES: Hirsutism, arched eyebrows, high-arched palate, congenital heart defects

ABNORMALITIES

Growth: Growth retardation

Performance: Hypotonia, mental retardation, convulsions

Eyes: Hypertelorism, arched eyebrows, epicanthal folds

Craniofacies: Ear malformations, hirsutism, low-set ears, synophrys, wide nasal bridge, anteverted nostrils, high-arched palate, thin upper lip, downturned corners of the mouth, micrognathia, short neck, long philtrum

Other: Congenital heart defects, clinodactyly, brachydactyly, bilateral simian creases, urogenital anomaly, limb anomalies

OCCASIONAL ABNORMALITIES: Undescended testes, widely spaced nipples.

CLINICAL COURSE: Survival into adulthood is common.

CYTOGENETICS: In many cases, chromosome 3q trisomy results from a parental chromosomal rearrangement.

REFERENCES

Aqua MS, Rizzu P, Lindsay EA, Shaffer LG, Zackai EH, Overhauser J, Baldini A. 1995. Duplication 3q syndrome: molecular delineation of the critical region. *Am. J. Med. Genet.* 55:33–37.

Chen CP, Liu FF, Jan SW, Chen CP, Lan CC. 1996. Partial duplication of 3q and distal deletion of 11q in a stillbirth with an omphalocele containing the liver, short limbs, and intrauterine growth retardation. *J. Med. Genet.* 33:615–617.

Holder SE, Grimsley LM, Palmer RW, Butler LJ, Baraitser M. 1994. Partial trisomy 3q causing mild Cornelia de Lange phenotype. *J. Med. Genet.* 31:150–152.

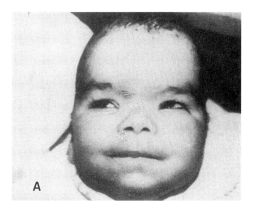 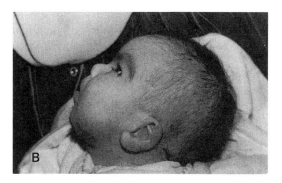

Note hypertelorism, hypertrichosis, long, prominent philtrum, and thin lips (a), short nose with anteverted nares, micrognathia, and apparently low-set, malformed ear (b). (From Ismail et al., 1991. *Am. J. Med. Genet.* 38:518–522. Copyright © 1991 John Wiley & Sons, Inc. Reprinted by permission of Wiley-Liss, Inc.)

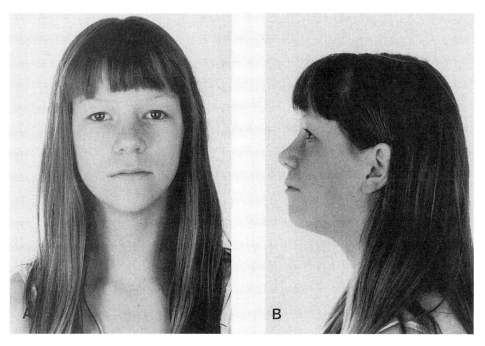

Patient at age 13 years. Note normal facial features. (From Lopez-Rangel et al., 1993. *Am. J. Med. Genet.* 47:1068–1071. Copyright © 1993 John Wiley & Sons, Inc. Reprinted by permission of Wiley-Liss, Inc.)

Ismail SR, Kousseff BG, Kotb SM, Kholeif SF. 1991. Duplication 3q(q21–qter) without limb anomalies. *Am. J. Med. Genet.* 38:518–522.

Lopez-Rangel E, Dill FJ, Hrynchak MA, Van Allen MI. 1993. Partial duplication of 3q(q25.1 → q26.1) without the Brachmann-de Lange phenotype. *Am. J. Med. Genet.* 47:1068–1071.

Rizzu P, Haddad BR, Vallcorba I, Alonso A, Ferro MT, Garcia-Sagredo JM, Baldini A. 1997. Delineation of a duplication map of chromosome 3q: a new case confirms the exclusion of 3q25–q26.2 from the duplication 3q syndrome critical region. *Am. J. Med. Genet.* 68:428–432.

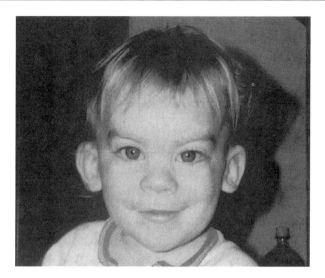

Note prominent, thickened, low-set, posteriorly angulated ears, epicanthus, synophrys, and anteverted nares. (From Aqua et al., 1995. *Am. J. Med. Genet.* 55:33–37. Copyright © 1995 John Wiley & Sons, Inc. Reprinted by permission of Wiley-Liss, Inc.)

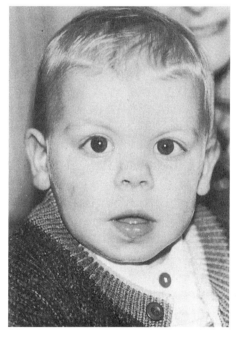

Patient at age 1 year and 4 months. Note arched eyebrows, epicanthic folds, flat nasal bridge, small, upturned nose, long philtrum, and thin upper lip. (From Holder et al., 1994. *J. Med. Genet.* 31:150–152. Reprinted with permission of BMJ Publishing Group.)

CHROMOSOME 3q PARTIAL MONOSOMY

Patients with deletions of 3q22 or 3q23 appear to have a distinctive phenotype. A majority of these deletions are de novo, resulting in a similar pattern of malformation.

MAIN FEATURES: Abnormal facial appearance, developmental delay, mental retardation

ABNORMALITIES

Performance: Mental retardation, developmental delay, psychomotor retardation, hypotonia

Craniofacies: Microcephaly, esotropia, nystagmus, blepharophimosis, ptosis, malformed ears, short palpebral fissures, synophrys, abnormal nose and nasal bridge, epicanthus inversus, epicanthal folds, abnormal mouth

Genitourinary: Cryptorchidism

Limbs: Tapering of the fingers, simian creases, joint contractures

Other: Respiratory distress

OCCASIONAL ABNORMALITIES: Cataracts, hypertelorism, hypertonia, scoliosis, heart defects

CLINICAL COURSE: Death in early infancy has been documented.

CYTOGENETICS: In almost all cases, the defects are de novo.

REFERENCES

Chitayat D, Babul R, Silver MM, Jay V, Teshima IE, Babyn P, Becker LE. 1996. Terminal deletion of the long arm of chromosome 3 [46,XX,del(3)(q27 → qter)]. *Am. J. Med. Genet.* 61:45–48.

Fujita H, Meng J, Kawamura M, Tozuka N, Ishii F, Tanaka N. 1992. Boy with a chromosome del(3)(q12q23) and blepharophimosis syndrome. *Am. J. Med. Genet.* 44:434–436.

Jewett T, Rao PN, Weaver RG, Stewart W, Thomas IT, Pettenati MJ. 1993. Blepharophimosis, ptosis, and epicanthus inversus syndrome (BPES) associated with interstitial deletion of band 3q22: review and gene assignment to the interface of band 3q22.3 and 3q23. *Am. J. Med. Genet.* 47:1147–1150.

Okada N, Hasegawa T, Osawa M, Fukuyama Y. 1987. A case of de novo interstitial deletion 3q. *J. Med. Genet.* 24:305–308.

Robin NH, Magnusson M, McDonald-McGinn D, Zackai EH, Spinner NB. 1993. De novo interstitial deletion of the long arm of chromosome 3: 46,XX,del(3)(q25.1q26.1). *Clin. Genet.* 44:335–337.

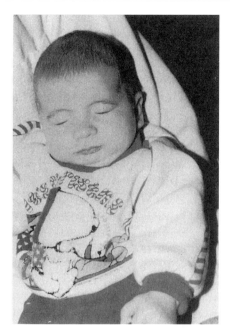

Patient at 2 months with eyes open. Note microcephaly, blepharophimosis with ptosis, and medial eyebrow flare. (From Jewett et al., 1993. *Am. J. Med. Genet.* 47:1147–1150. Copyright © 1993 John Wiley & Sons, Inc. Reprinted by permission of Wiley-Liss, Inc.)

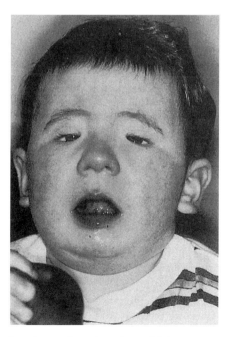

Patient at 1 year and 9 months of age after elevation of lids. Note prominent epicanthus inversus bilaterally is present. (From Jewett et al., 1993. *Am. J. Med. Genet.* 47:1147–1150. Copyright © 1993 John Wiley & Sons, Inc. Reprinted by permission of Wiley-Liss, Inc.)

RING CHROMOSOME 3

Patients with ring chromosome 3 are extremely rare. Due to the small number of patients with this defect, it is not possible to identify a distinctive syndrome.

MAIN FEATURES: Microcephaly, growth retardation, develpmental delay

ABNORMALITIES

Growth: Growth retardation

Performance: Developmental delay

Craniofacies: Microcephaly, small anterior fontanelle, synophrys, bushy eyebrows, low anterior hairline

Genitourinary: Genital abnormalities

Other: Heart murmur

CLINICAL COURSE: Survival into late childhood has been documented.

CYTOGENETICS: Reported patients are the result of a de novo defect.

REFERENCES

Lakshminarayana P, Nallasivam P. 1990. Cornelia de Lange syndrome with ring chromosome 3. *J. Med. Genet.* 27:405–406.

Yip MY, MacKenzie H, Kovacic A, McIntosh A. 1996. Chromosome 3p23 break with ring formation and translocation of displaced 3p23 → pter segment to 6pter. *J. Med. Genet.* 33:789–792.

CHROMOSOME 4p PARTIAL TRISOMY

Patients with partial duplications of 4p generally exhibit a variable phenpotype. Several features are distinctive findings of 4p partial trisomy, including large, simple ears and a bulbous nose. Generally, these patients result from a parental chromosomal rearrangement, which contributes to the variation of phenotypes.

MAIN FEATURES: Large, simple ears, bulbous nose, short neck

ABNORMALITIES

Growth: Growth retardation

Performance: Developmental delay, mental retardation, psychomotor retardation, failure to thrive

Craniofacies: Microcephaly, abnormally shaped head, short neck, large, simple ears, high palate, small, triangular mouth, bulbous nose

Limbs: Short, broad hands and feet

Other: Low anterior hairline, widely spaced nipples

OCCASIONAL ABNORMALITIES: Long, receding chin, cardiac defects, hypotonia

CLINICAL COURSE: Suvival into adulthood is not uncommon.

CYTOGENETICS: Most patients result from parental chromosomal rearrangements, but de novo defects have been reported.

REFERENCES

Hastings R, Hamer B, Roth S, Lucas M. 1990. Partial trisomy 4p resulting from a balanced intrachromosomal insertion, 4(q313p14p16). *Clin. Genet.* 38:121–125.

Kleczkowska A, Fryns JP, van den Berghe H. 1992. Trisomy of the short arm of chromosome 4: the changing phenotype with age. *Ann. Genet.* 35:217-223.

Oorthuys JW, Gerssen-Schoorl KB, de Pater JM, de France HF. 1989. A third case of de novo partial trisomy 4p. *J. Med. Genet.* 26:344–345.

Wyandt HE, Milunsky J, Lerner T, Gusella JF, Hou A, MacDonald M, Adekunle S, Milunsky A. 1993. Characterization of a duplication in the terminal band of 4p by molecular cytogenetics. *Am. J. Med. Genet.* 46:72–76.

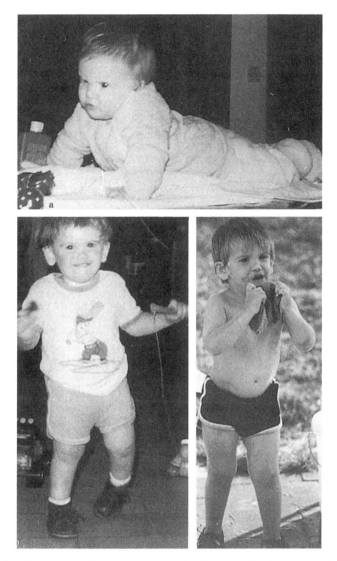

Patient at 6 months, 2 years and 3 years respectively. Note small, sloping forehead, protruding supraorbital ridges, low anterior hairline, sparse eyelashes and eyebrows, downward-slanting palpebral fissures, ptosis, bilateral epicanthal folds, flat midface, broad, depressed nasal bridge, bulbous nasal tip, triangular mouth, long philtrum, thin lips, and chubby cheeks and clenched hands. (From Kleczkowska et al., 1992. *Ann. Genet.* 4:217–223. Reprinted with permission of Expansion Scientifique Francaise.)

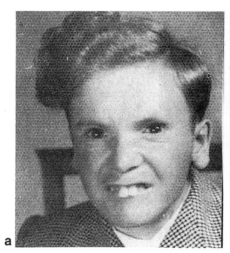
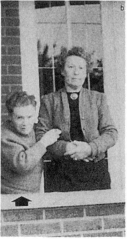

Patient at 20 and 36 years respectively. Note prominent supraorbital ridges, deeply set eyes, downward-slanting palpebral fissures, bilateral epicanthal folds, broad nasal bridge, and fine lips. (From Kleczkowska et al., 1992. *Ann. Genet.* 4:217–223. Reprinted with permission of Expansion Scientifique Francaise.)

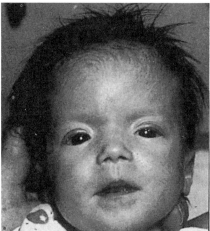
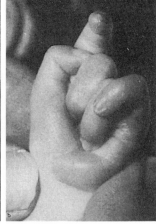

Patient at 3 months. Note small, sloping forehead, protruding supraorbital ridges, low anterior hairline, sparse eyelashes and eyebrows, downward-slanting palpebral fissures, ptosis, epicanthal folds, broad, depressed nasal bridge, bulbous nasal tip, triangular mouth, long philtrum, thin lips, and chubby cheeks (a) and clenched hand with overlapping fingers and camptodactyly (b). (From Kleczkowska et al., 1992. *Ann. Genet.* 4:217–223. Reprinted with permission of Expansion Scientifique Francaise.)

CHROMOSOME 4p PARTIAL MONOSOMY

Partial deletion for the short arm of chromosome 4 is also known as Wolf-Hirschbolm syndrome (WHS). The defect can involve most of the short arm of chromosome 4. However, the critical region appears to be located in region p16.

MAIN FEATURES: Mental retardation, prominent forehead

ABNORMALITIES

Growth: Prenatal growth deficiency

Performance: Mental retardation, developmental delay, psychomotor retardation, seizures, hypotonia

Eyes: Hypertelorism, strabismus, iris deformities

Craniofacies: Microcephaly, craniofacial deformities, prominent glabella (forehead), broad nasal bridge, epicanthal folds, downturned fishlike mouth, cleft lip/palate, short or long philtrum, micrognathia, ear malformations, abnormal nose

Other: Abnormal dermatoglyphics, cryptorchidism

CLINICAL COURSE: These patients exhibit growth and developmental delays. If there are no significant physical defects, survival into adulthood is possible.

CYTOGENETICS: In most instances, the patient represents a de novo defect, although parental chromosomal rearrangements do occur.

REFERENCES

Chitayat D, Ruvalcaba RH, Babul R, Teshima IE, Posnick JC, Vekemans MJ, Scarpelli H, Thuline H. 1995. Syndrome of proximal interstitial deletion 4p15: report of three cases and review of the literature. *Am. J. Med. Genet.* 55:147–154.

Clemens M, Martsolf JT, Rogers JG, Mowery-Rushton P, Surti U, McPherson E. 1996. Pitt-Rogers-Danks syndrome: the result of a 4p microdeletion. *Am. J. Med. Genet.* 66:95–100.

Davies J, Voullaire L, Bankier A. 1990. Interstitial deletion of the band 4p15.3 defined by sequential replication banding. *Ann. Genet.* 33:92–95.

Fryns JP. 1995. Syndrome of proximal interstitial deletion 4p15. *Am. J. Med. Genet.* 58:295–296.

Fryns JP, Yang-Aisheng, Kleczkowska A, Lemmens F, Vandecasseye W, van den Berghe H. 1989. Interstitial deletion of the short arm of chromosome 4. A phenotype distinct from the Wolf-Hirschhorn syndrome. *Ann. Genet.* 32:59–61.

Phelan MC, Saul RA, Gailey TA Jr, Skinner SA. 1995. Prenatal diagnosis of mosaic 4p- in a fetus with trisomy 21. *Prenat. Diagn.* 15:274–277.

Vockley J, Inserra JA, Breg WR, Yang-Feng TL. 1991. "Pseudomosaicism" for 4p- in amniotic fluid cell culture proven to be true mosaicism after birth. *Am. J. Med. Genet.* 39:81–83.

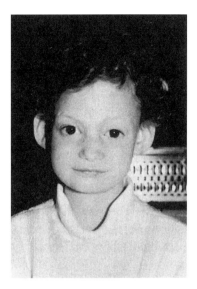

Patient at age 7 years and 9 months. Note short facial height, wide mouth, short philtrum, maxillary hypoplasia, short mandible, slightly beaked nose, simple, low-set, prominent ears. (From Clemens et al., 1996. *Am. J. Med. Genet.* 66:95–100. Copyright © 1996 John Wiley & Sons, Inc. Reprinted by permission of Wiley-Liss, Inc.)

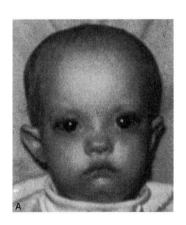 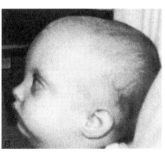 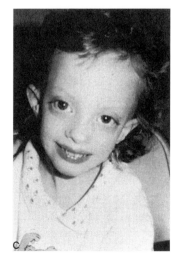

Patient at age 5 months (A,B) and 4 years and 8 months (C). Note prominent forehead, proptotic eyes, hypoplastic maxilla, micrognathia, and relatively large ears. From Clemens et al., 1996. *Am. J. Med. Genet.* 66:95–100. Copyright © 1996 John Wiley & Sons, Inc. Reprinted by permission of Wiley-Liss, Inc.)

CHROMOSOME 4q PARTIAL TRISOMY

Patients with partial trisomy for different segments 4q exhibit variable phenotypes. Individuals with trisomy of the distal third of chromosome 4q present with a predictable pattern of manifestations (see below), including growth and psychomotor retardation.

MAIN FEATURES: Growth and psychomotor retardation, low-set, abnormal ears, and microcephaly

ABNORMALITIES

Growth: Growth retardation

Performance: Psychomotor retardation, mental retardation, hypotonia

Craniofacies: Microcephaly, abnormal, low-set ears, short neck, abnormal palpebral fissures, epicanthal folds, abnormal nasal bridge, long philtrum, carplike mouth, thick, protruding lips

Limbs: Limb movement deficiencies, rigidity of joints, abnormal fingers and toes

Other: Hirsutism

OCCASIONAL ABNORMALITIES: Ptosis, synophrys, tetralogy of Fallot, seizures

CLINICAL COURSE: Survival into adulthood has been documented.

CYTOGENETICS: In most instances, the patient results from a parental chromosomal rearrangement, although de novo defects do occur.

REFERENCES

de Almeida JC, Reis DF, Llerena Junior JC. 1991. Pure 4p trisomy due to a de novo 4q;22p dicentric translocated chromosome karyotype 46,XX,-22,+t(4;22)(q1200;p13). *Ann. Genet.* 34:108–110.

Halal F, Vekemans M, Chitayat D. 1991. Interstitial tandem direct duplication of the long arm of chromosome 4(q23–q27) and possible assignment of the structural gene encoding human aspartylglucosaminidase to this segment. *Am. J. Med. Genet.* 39:418–421.

Mikelsaar RV, Lurie IW, Ilus TE. 1996. "Pure" partial trisomy 4q25-qter owing to a de novo 4;22 translocation. *J. Med. Genet.* 33:344–345.

Navarro EG, Romero MC, Exposito IL, Velasco CM, Llamas JG, Ramon FJ, Jimenez RD. 1996. De novo interstitial tandem duplication of chromosome 4(q21–q28). *Am. J. Med. Genet.* 62:297–299.

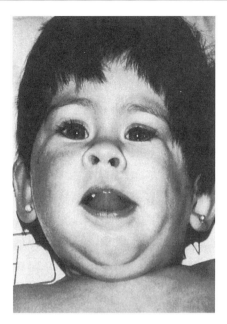

Note facial asymmetry, upward-slanting, short palepebral fissures, hypotelorism, bilateral epicanthal folds, slightly enlarged auricles, high nasal bridge, upturned nose, long, pronounced philtrum, micrognathia, protruding lower lip, and short neck. (From Navarro et al., 1996. *Am. J. Med. Genet.* 62:297–299. Copyright © 1996 John Wiley & Sons, Inc. Reprinted by permission of Wiley-Liss, Inc.)

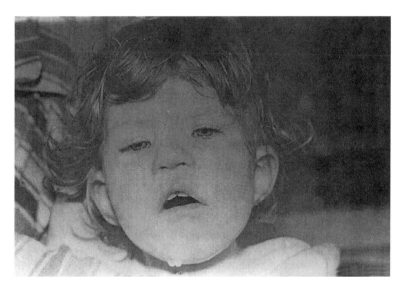

Patient at 1 year and 6 months. Note epicanthal folds, slightly downward-slanting palpebral fissures, left-sided ptosis, prominent nasal bridge, protruding upper lip, short philtrum, large, low-set, malformed ears, and short neck. (From Mikelsaar et al., 1995. *J. Med. Genet.* 33:344–345. Reprinted with permission from BMJ Publishing Group.)

CHROMOSOME 4q PARTIAL MONOSOMY

Patients with interstitial deletions of 4q are rare and do not exhibit a predictable phenotype. However, patients with terminal deletions of 4q are much more common. These individuals usually present with characteristic features, including, micrognathia and develpmental delay (see below).

MAIN FEATURES: Micrognathia, malformed ears, developmental delay

ABNORMALITIES

Growth: Short stature

Performance: Developmental delay, mental retardation, hypotonia

Craniofacies: Large anterior fontanelle, frontal bossing, malformed, low-set ears, abnormal palpebral fissures, short nose, flat nasal bridge, upward-slanting eyes, high, narrow palate, micrognathia, small teeth

Limbs: Short limbs, clinodactyly of the fifth finger, and abnormal fingers toes

Other: Sparse hair, widely spaced nipples

OCCASIONAL ABNORMALITIES: Cardiac defects, seizures, and psychomotor retardation

CLINICAL COURSE: Most reported patients have been children. Life expectancy is unknown.

CYTOGENETICS: In most instances, the patient represents a de novo defect although parental chromosomal rearrangements do occur.

REFERENCES

Copelli S, del Rey G, Heinrich J, Coco R. 1995. Brief clinical report: interstitial deletion of the long arm of chromosome 4, del(4)(q28 → q31.3). *Am. J. Med. Genet.* 55:77–79.

Hegmann KM, Spikes AS, Orr-Urtreger A, Shaffer LG. 1996. Segregation of a paternal insertional translocation results in partial 4q monosomy or 4q trisomy in two siblings. *Am. J. Med. Genet.* 61:10–15.

Kulharya AS, Maberry M, Kukolich MK, Day DW, Schneider NR, Wilson GN, Tonk V. 1995. Interstitial deletions 4q21.1q25 and 4q25q27: phenotypic variability and relation to Rieger anomaly. *Am. J. Med. Genet.* 55:165–170.

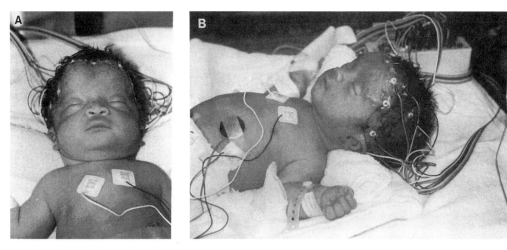

Note frontal bossing, facial hirsutism, flat supraorbital ridges, short nose, and apparently low-set, posteriorly angulated ears. (From Kulharya et al., *Am. J. Med. Genet.* 55:165–170. Copyright © 1995 John Wiley & Sons, Inc. Reprinted by permission of Wiley-Liss, Inc.)

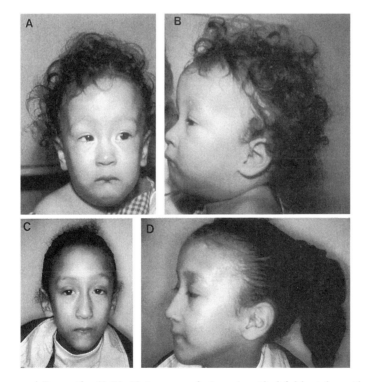

Patient at 1 year and 7 months (A,B). Note sparse hair, epicanthal folds, telecanthus, flat supraorbital ridges, flat nasal bridge, small nose, upturned nostrils, down-curved mouth, and thin lower lip. Patient at 9 years and 6 months (C,D). Note bilateral ptosis, upward-slanting palpebral fissures, high nasal bridge, and small down-curved mouth with thin lips. (From Kulharya et al., *Am. J. Med. Genet.* 55:165–170. Copyright © 1995 John Wiley & Sons, Inc. Reprinted by permission of Wiley-Liss, Inc.)

Menko FH, Madan K, Baart JA, Beukenhorst HL. 1992. Robin sequence and a deficiency of the left forearm in a girl with a deletion of chromosome 4q33-qter. *Am. J. Med. Genet.* 44:696–698.

Rose NC, Schneider A, McDonald-McGinn DM, Caserta C, Emanuel BS, Zackai EH. 1991. Interstitial deletion of 4(q21q25) in a liveborn male. *Am. J. Med. Genet.* 40:77–79.

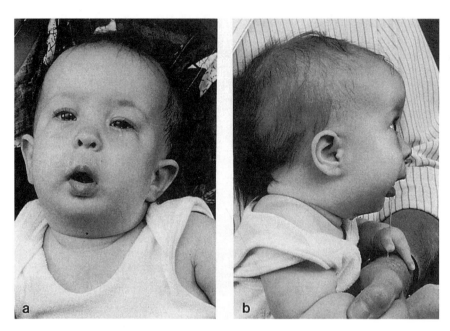

Note flat nasal bridge, slight upward slant of the eyes, and micrognathia. (From Menko et al., 1992. *Am. J. Med. Genet.* 44:696–698. Copyright © 1992 John Wiley & Sons, Inc. Reprinted by permission of Wiley-Liss, Inc.)

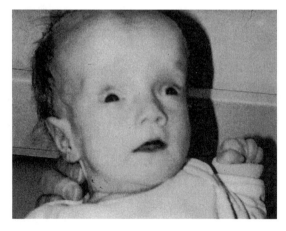

Patient at 7 weeks. Note prominent frontal bossing, hypertelorism, small palpebral fissures, upward-slanting eyes, micrognathia, flat nasal bridge, and short, malformed philtrum. (From Rose et al., 1991. *Am. J. Med. Genet.* 40:77–79. Copyright © 1991 John Wiley & Sons, Inc. Reprinted by permission of Wiley-Liss, Inc.)

RING CHROMOSOME 4

Patients with ring chromosome 4 are relatively rare. These patients present with different amounts of chromosome 4 deleted, but all exhibit some degree of malformation.

MAIN FEATURES: Microcephaly, intrauterine growth retardation (IUGR), severe growth retardation, mental retardation

ABNORMALITIES

Growth: IUGR, severe growth retardation

Performance: Mental retardation

Craniofacies: Microcephaly, micrognathia, beaked nose, short philtrum, large ears

Limbs: Clinodactyly

Other: Cardiac defects

OCCASIONAL ABNORMALITIES: Hypertelorism, ptosis, hypospadius, cryptorchidism

CLINICAL COURSE: Death in infancy is not uncommon.

CYTOGENETICS: Reported patients are the result of a de novo defect.

REFERENCES

Bobrow M, Joness LF, Clarke G. 1971. A complex chromosomal rearrangement with formation of a ring 4. *J. Med. Genet.* 8:235–239.

Halal F, Vekemans M, Kaplan P, Zeesman S. 1990. Distal deletion of chromosome 1q in an adult. *Am. J. Med. Genet.* 37:79–82.

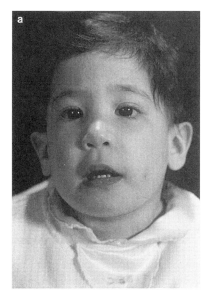
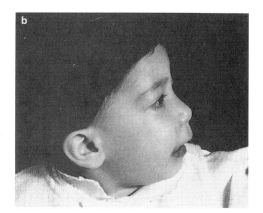

Note mild epicanthal folds, prominent ears with slightly hypoplastic helices, depressed nasal bridge, long philtrum, and mild retromicrognathia. (From Halal and Vekemans, 1990. *Am. J. Med. Genet.* 37:79–82. Copyright © 1990 John Wiley & Sons, Inc. Reprinted by permission of Wiley-Liss, Inc.)

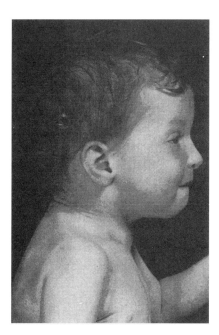
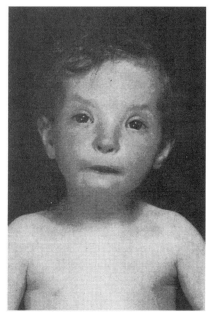

Patient at 2 years. Note hypertelorism, bilateral epicanthus, micrognathia, overhanging upper lip, slightly low-set ears, and widely spaced nipples. (From Bobrow et al., 1971. *J. Med. Genet.* 8:235–239. Reprinted with permission from BMJ Publishing Group.)

CHROMOSOME 5p PARTIAL TRISOMY

Partial duplications of 5p produces patients with some similarities. One patient with partial trisomy of 5p had features similar to the Opitz BBBG syndrome.

MAIN FEATURES: Broad/deep nasal bridge, abnormal skull shape, low-set ears, microretrognathia

ABNORMALITIES

Growth: Growth retardation, failure to thrive, developmental delay, short stature

Performance: Respiratory distress, seizures, hypotonia, psychomotor retardation

Craniofacies: Abnormal scull shape, broad/deep nasal bridge, microretrognathia, macrocephaly, ear malformations, abnormal palpebral fissures, hypertelorism, epicanthal folds, macroglossia, low-set dysplastic ears

Other: Clubfoot, cryptorchidism, arachnodactyly, congenital heart defect

CLINICAL COURSE: Early death is common.

CYTOGENETICS: Most patients result from a parental chromosomal rearrangement.

REFERENCES

Chen H, Hoffman WH, Kusyk CJ, Tuck-Muller CM, Hoffman MG, Davis LS. 1995. De novo dup (5p) in a patient with congenital hypoplasia of the adrenal gland. *Am. J. Med. Genet.* 55:489–493.

Leichtman LG, Werner A, Bass WT, Smith D, Brothman AR. 1991. Apparent Opitz BBBG syndrome with a partial duplication of 5p. *Am. J. Med. Genet.* 40:173–176.

Lorda-Sanchez I, Urioste M, Villa A, Carrascosa MC, Vazquez MS, Martinez A, Martinez-Frias ML. 1997. Proximal partial 5p trisomy resulting from a maternal (19;5) insertion. *Am. J. Med. Genet.* 68:476–480.

Qumsiyeh MB, Stevens CA. 1993. Two sibs with different phenotypes due to adjacent-1 segregation of a subtle translocation t(4;5)(p16.3;p15.3)mat. *Am. J. Med. Genet.* 47:387–391.

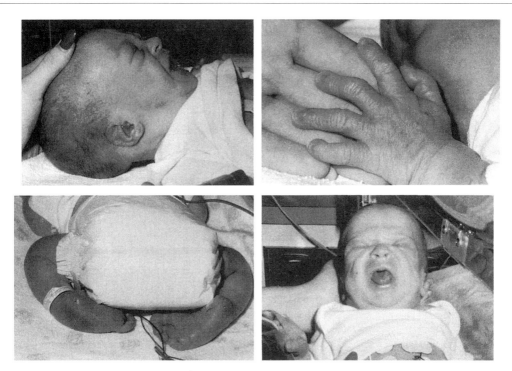

Note low-set ears, clinodactyly, arachnodactyly, talipes equinovarus, and hypertelorism. (From Leichtman et al., 1991. *Am. J. Med. Genet.* 40:173–176. Copyright © 1991 John Wiley & Sons, Inc. Reprinted by permission of Wiley-Liss, Inc.)

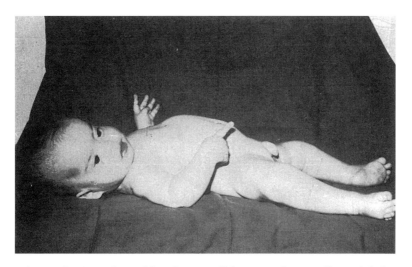

Patient at age 6 months. Note frontal bossing, small low-set, abnormally modeled ears, mild epicanthus, flat nasal bridge, hypertelorism, short nose, midface hypoplasia, full lips, and micrognathia. (From Lorda-Sánchez et al., 1997. *Am. J. Med. Genet.* 68:476–480. Copyright © 1997 John Wiley & Sons, Inc. Reprinted by permission of Wiley-Liss, Inc.)

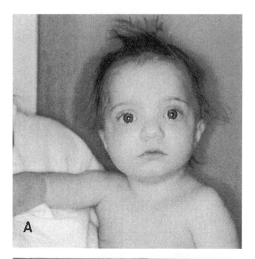

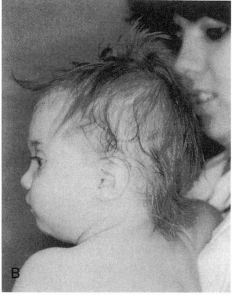

Patient at age 1 year and 6 months. Note unruly hair, long eyelashes, broad nasal bridge, well-defined philtrum, and downturned mouth. (From Qumsiyeh and Stevens, 1993. *Am. J. Med. Genet.* 47:387–391. Copyright © 1993 John Wiley & Sons, Inc. Reprinted by permission of Wiley-Liss, Inc.)

CHROMOSOME 5p PARTIAL MONOSOMY
Cri-du-chat Syndrome

Patients with deletions of 5p, including the band 5p15.2, exhibit cri-du-chat syndrome. It appears that this deletion is present in all patients with this syndrome. Deletions of 5p that do not contain the critical band of 5p15.2 result in a clinically variable phenotypes.

MAIN FEATURES: Developmental delay, malformed ears, microcephaly

ABNORMALITIES

Performance: Developmental delay, mental retardation, hypertonia, and poor feeding

Craniofacies: Malformed, low-set ears, microcephaly, downward-slanting palpebral fissures, abnormal nose, broad nasal bridge, epicanthal folds, high-arched palate, hypertelorism, and thin lips

Limbs: Clinodacyly and long fingers

Other: Inguinal hernia

OCCASIONAL ABNORMALITIES: Short stature, simian creases, limb abnormalities, and hypotonia

CLINICAL COURSE: Survival into adulthood is not uncommon.

CYTOGENETICS: Most patients result from parental chromosomal rearrangements, but de novo defects have been reported.

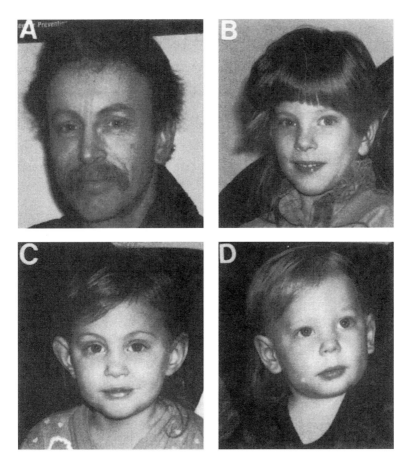

Family with inherited deletion (From Gersh et al., 1995. *Am. J. Hum. Genet.* 56:1404–1410. Copyright © 1995 The University of Chicago Press. Reprinted by permission.)

REFERENCES

Gersh M, Goodart SA, Pasztor LM, Harris DJ, Weiss L, Overhauser J. 1995. Evidence for a distinct region causing a cat-like cry in patients with 5p deletions. *Am. J. Hum. Genet.* 56:1404–1410.

Keppen LD, Gollin SM, Edwards D, Sawyer J, Wilson W, Overhauser J. 1992. Clinical phenotype and molecular analysis of a three-generation family with an interstitial deletion of the short arm of chromosome 5. *Am. J. Med. Genet.* 44:356–360.

Schuffenhauer S, Kobelt A, Daumer-Haas C, Loffler C, Muller G, Murken J, Meitinger T. 1996. Interstitial deletion 5p accompanied by dicentric ring formation of the deleted segment resulting in trisomy 5p13-cen. *Am. J. Med. Genet.* 65:56–59.

Szego K, Rauer M, Baratta E, Hoo JJ. 1993. De novo concurrent 5p deletion and distal 17q duplication identified by fluorescence in situ hybridization (FISH). *Ann. Genet.* 36:224–227.

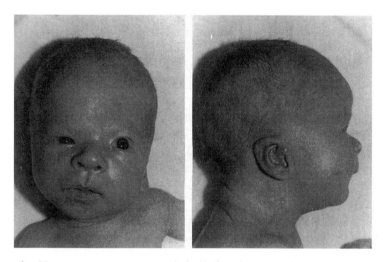

Patient at 2 weeks. Note square asymmetrical skull, facial asymmetry, hypertelorism, epicanthal folds, short, broad nose, broad, flat nasal bridge, long, deep philtrum, microretrognathia, low-set, abnormally modeled ears. (From Schuffenhauer et al., 1996. *Am. J. Med. Genet.* 65:56–59. Copyright © 1996 John Wiley & Sons, Inc. Reprinted by permission of Wiley-Liss, Inc.)

CHROMOSOME 5q PARTIAL TRISOMY

There appears to be some similar features in the few patients with partial duplication of the long arm of chromosome 5. Bassett et al. (1988) and McGillivray et al. (1990) theorized that a gene for schizophrenia is located around 5q11.2–q13.3. Two 5q+ patients have so far been diagnosed with schizophrenia.

MAIN FEATURES: Craniosynostosis, congenital heart defect, renal anomalies

ABNORMALITIES

Growth: Growth retardation

Performance: Mental retardation, hypotonia

Craniofacies: Craniosynostosis, prominent forehead, ear abnormalities, low-set ears, abnormal palpebral fissures, hypertelorism wide nasal bridge, epicanthus, short neck

Other: Congenital heart defect, respiratory distress, renal anomalies

CLINICAL COURSE: Death in the newborn period has been noted.

CYTOGENETICS: Frequently resulting from a parental chromosomal rearrangement.

REFERENCES

Bassett AS, McGillivray BC, Jones BD, Pantzar JT. 1988. Partial trisomy chromosome 5 cosegregating with schizophrenia. *Lancet.* 1:799–801.

Breslau-Siderius EJ, Wijnen JT, Dauwerse JG, de Pater JM, Beemer FA, Khan PM. 1993. Paternal duplication of chromosome 5q11.2–5q14 in a male born with craniostenosis, ear tags, kidney dysplasia and several other anomalies. *Hum. Genet.* 92:481–485.

Lai MM, Scriven PN, Ball C, Berry AC. 1992. Simultaneous partial monosomy 10p and trisomy 5q in a case of hypoparathyroidism. *J. Med. Genet.* 29:586–588.

McGillivray BC, Bassett AS, Langlois S, Pantzar T, Wood S. 1990. Familial 5q11.2–q13.3 segmental duplication cosegregating with multiple anomalies, including schizophrenia. *Am. J. Med. Genet.* 35:10–13.

Schimmenti LA, Higgins RR, Mendelsohn NJ, Casey TM, Steinberger J, Mammel MC, Wiesner GL. 1995. Monosomy 9p24 → pter and trisomy 5q31 → qter: case report and review of two cases. *Am. J. Med. Genet.* 57:52–56.

Van Der Burgt CJ, Merkx GF, Janssen AH, Mulder JC, Suijkerbuijk RF, Smeets DF. 1992. Partial trisomy for 5q and monosomy for 12p in a liveborn child as a result of a complex five breakpoint chromosome rearrangement in a parent. *J. Med. Genet.* 29:739–741.

Yip MY, Kemp J, Hanson N, Wilson M, Purvis-Smith S, Lam-Po-Tang PR. 1989. Duplication of 5q11.2–q13.1 from a familial (5;20) balanced insertion. *Am. J. Med. Genet.* 33:220–223.

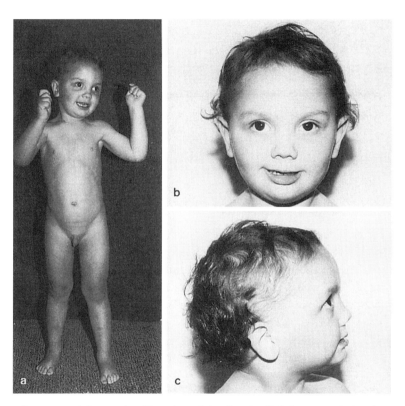

Patient at age 2 years and 9 months. Note broad forehead, slightly upward-slanting palpebral fissures, scattered eyebrows, hypertelorism, wide, flat nasal bridge, slightly anteverted nares, flat facial profile, and slightly upturned corners of the mouth. (From Yip et al., 1989. *Am. J. Med. Genet.* 32:220–223. Copyright © 1989 John Wiley & Sons, Inc. Reprinted by permission of Wiley-Liss, Inc.)

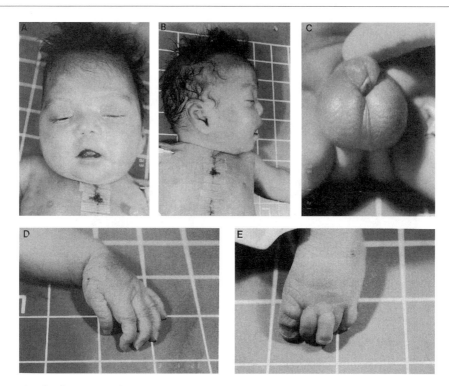

Patient at birth after 33 weeks gestation. Note face demonstrating low frontal hairline, abnormal philtrum, and broad nasal bridge (A). Profile demonstrating apparently low-set ears (B). Genitalia of infant with hypospadias and bifid scrotum (C). Hand of infant with triphalangeal thumb (D). Foot of infant with 2–3 syndactyly and third toe overlapping fourth toe (E). (From Schimmenti et al., 1995. *Am. J. Med. Genet.* 57:52–56. Copyright © 1995 John Wiley & Sons, Inc. Reprinted by permission of Wiley-Liss, Inc.)

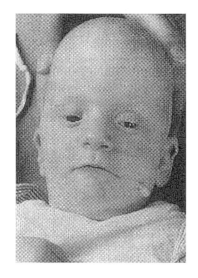

Patient at age 5 months. Note long, narrow skull, prominent forehead, skin tags, mouth with downturned corners. (From Breslau-Siderius et al., 1993. *Hum. Genet.* 92:481–485. Copyright © 1993 Springer-Verlag. Reprinted with permission.)

CHROMOSOME 5q PARTIAL MONOSOMY

Deletions that span 5q21 → q22 will include the adenomatous polyposis coli (APC) gene, which is involved in familial adenomatous polyposis (FAP) and sporadic colon cancer. Therefore, this is one of the main characteristics of these patients.

MAIN FEATURES: Adenomata/polyposis, prominaent forehead, ear malformations, mental retardation

ABNORMALITIES

Growth: Failure to thrive

Performance: Mild to profound mental retardation, developmental delay, poor feeding, hypotonia

Eyes: Hypertelorism, eye abnormalities, congenital hypertrophy of the retinal pigmentary epithelium (CHRPE)

Craniofacies: Prominent forehead, ear malformations, flat and broad nasal bridge, long midface, anteverted nostrils, high-arched palate, prominent jaw, macrognathia

Other: Adenomata polyposis, carcinoma of the colon/rectum, subcutaneous lesions, abnormal chest shape, dislocated hips

CLINICAL COURSE: Life into adulthood is common.

CYTOGENETICS: De novo and resulting from a familial chromosomal translocation.

REFERENCES

Barber JC, Ellis KH, Bowles LV, Delhanty JD, Ede RF, Male BM, Eccles DM. 1994. Adenomatous polyposis coli and a cytogenetic deletion of chromosome 5 resulting from a maternal intrachromosomal insertion. *J. Med. Genet.* 31:312–316.

Cross I, Delhanty J, Chapman P, Bowles LV, Griffin D, Wolstenholme J, Bradburn M, Brown J, Wood C, Gunn A, et al. 1992. An intrachromosomal insertion causing 5q22 deletion and familial adenomatous polyposis coli in two generations. *J. Med. Genet.* 29:175–179.

Hodgson SV, Coonar AS, Hanson PJ, Cottrell S, Scriven PN, Jones T, Hawley PR, Wilkinson ML. 1993. Two cases of 5q deletions in patients with familial adenomatous polyposis: possible link with Caroli's disease. *J. Med. Genet.* 30:369–375.

Kleczkowska A, Fryns JP, van den Berghe H. 1993. A distinct multiple congenital anomalies syndrome associated with distal 5q deletion (q35.1qter). *Ann. Genet.* 36:126–128.

Lindgren V, Bryke CR, Ozcelik T, Yang-Feng TL, Francke U. 1992. Phenotypic, cytogenetic, and molecular studies of three patients with constitutional deletions of chromosome 5 in the region of the gene for familial adenomatous polyposis. *Am. J. Hum. Genet.* 50:988–997.

Stratton RF, Tedrowe NA, Tolworthy JA, Patterson RM, Ryan SG, Young RS. 1994. Deletion 5q35.3. *Am. J. Med. Genet.* 51:150–152.

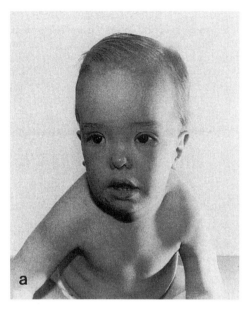

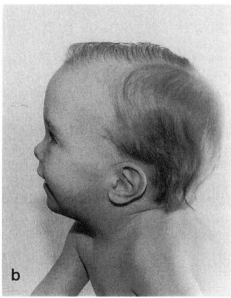

Patient at age 1 year and 3 months. Note redundant nuchal skin, telecanthus, flat nasal bridge, anteverted nares, retrognathia, and bell-shaped chest. (From Stratton et al., 1994. *Am. J. Med. Genet.* 51:150–152. Copyright © 1994 John Wiley & Sons, Inc. Reprinted by permission of Wiley-Liss, Inc.)

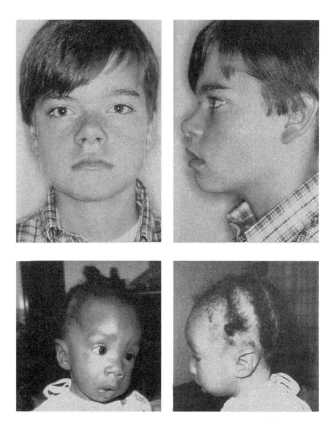

Top: Patient 1 at age 13 years. Note prominent forehead, hypertelorism, depressed nasal bridge, bulbous nose, anteverted nares, wide philtrum, prognathism, cupid's bow-shaped upper lip. Bottom: Patient 2 at age 8 months. Note biparietal prominence, high prominent forehead, hypoplastic supraorbital ridges, hypertelorism, downward-slanting palpebral fissures, epicanthal folds, broad flat nasal bridge, anteverted nares, long, poorly defined philtrum, small mouth, micrognathia, and short neck. (From Lindgren et al., 1992. *Am. J. Hum. Genet.* 50:988–997. Copyright © 1992 The University of Chicago Press. Reprinted with permission.)

RING CHROMOSOME 5

Ring chromosome 5 is an extremely rare finding. If ring formation results in the loss of 5q21 → q22, the patient should manifest familial adenomatous polyposis (FAP). Other patients will exhibit "ring syndrome," which leads to severe growth failure as the major feature. Rings resulting in the loss of a portion of 5q may result in additional dysmorphic features.

MAIN FEATURES: Unusual facial appearance, severe growth retardation, and failure to thrive

ABNORMALITIES

Growth: Severe growth retardation

Performance: Poor feeding, failure to thrive, and hypotonia

Craniofacies: Unusual facial features, including microcephaly, narrow forehead, downward-slanting palpebral fissures, prominent nasal bridge, hypertelorism, micrognathia, deep philtrum, and downturned mouth

Limbs: Abnormal fingers

Other: Cardiac defects

CLINICAL COURSE: Survival into childhood is documented.

CYTOGENETICS: Reported patients are the result of a de novo defect.

REFERENCES

Flannery DB, Rogers WG, Byrd JR. 1988. Ring chromosome 5. *Clin. Genet.* 34:74–78.

Migliori MV, Cherubini V, Bartolotta E, Pettinari A, Pecora R. 1994. Ring chromosome 5 associated with severe growth retardation as the sole major physical abnormality. *Am. J. Med. Genet.* 49:108–110.

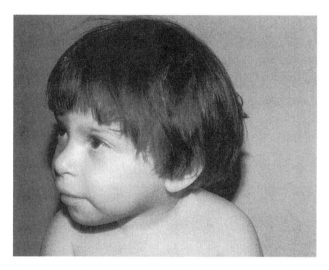

Patient at 3 years. Note short neck and near-normal facial appearance. (From Migliori et al., 1994. *Am. J. Med. Genet.* 49:108–110. Copyright © 1994 John Wiley & Sons, Inc. Reprinted by permission of Wiley-Liss, Inc.)

CHROMOSOME 6p PARTIAL TRISOMY

Patients with partial trisomy for 6p are relatively rare. Most often, these defects arise from parental chromosomal rearrangements. These patients generally present with a predictable pattern of malformation.

MAIN FEATURES: Malformed, low-set ears, growth retardation, and developmental delay

ABNORMALITIES

Growth: Low birth weight, growth retardation

Performance: Developmental delay, mental retardation, psychomotor retardation, poor feeding

Craniofacies: Malformed, low-set ears, high forehead, abnormal sutures, ptosis, blepharoptosis, blepharophimosis

Other: Abnormal lungs and/or pulmonary function

OCCASIONAL ABNORMALITIES: Microcephaly, downward-slanting palpebral fissures, long philtrum, thin lips, small pointed chin, thin sparse hair, abnormal fingers and toes

CLINICAL COURSE: Death in childhood is not uncommon.

CYTOGENETICS: Most patients result from parental chromosomal rearrangements, but de novo defects have been reported.

REFERENCES

Cote GB, Papadakou-Lagoyanni S, Sbyrakis S. 1978. Partial trisomy 6p with karyotype 46,XY,der(22),(6;22)(p22;q13mat. *J. Med. Genet.* 15:479–481.

Eden MS, Thelin JW, Michalski K, Mitchell JA. 1985. Partial trisomy 6p and partial monosomy 9p from a de novo translocation 46,XY,-9,+Der(9)T(6:9)(p211:p24). *Clin. Genet.* 28:375–384.

Fryns JP, Kleczkowska A, Moerman F, van den Berghe K, van den Berghe H. 1986. Partial distal 6p trisomy in a malformed fetus. *Ann. Genet.* 29:53–54.

Scarbrough PR, Carroll AJ, Finley SC, Hamerick K. 1986. Partial trisomy 6p and partial trisomy 22 resulting from 3:1 meiotic disjunction of maternal (6p;22q) translocation. *J. Med. Genet.* 23:185–187.

CHROMOSOME 6p PARTIAL MONOSOMY

Patients with partial deletions of 6p are relatively rare. Generally, these individuals result from a de novo loss of genetic material and present with some predictable features.

MAIN FEATURES: Malformed, low-set ears, abnormal sutures, and mental retardation

ABNORMALITIES

Performance: Developmental delay, mental retardation, psychomotor retardation, hypotonia

Craniofacies: Malformed, low-set ears, microcephaly, abnormal sutures, short neck, abnormal palpebral fissures, broad nasal bridge, abnormal nose and philtrum, micrognathia

Genitourinary: Genital abnormalities

Limbs: Abnormal hands and feet with abnormal fingers and toes

Other: Highly arched palate, patent ductus arteriosus, other cardiac defects

OCCASIONAL ABNORMALITIES: Hydrocephalus, large anterior fontanelle, epicanthal folds, cleft lip and palate, umbilical hernia, clinodactyly, simian crease, growth retardation, and widely spaced nipples

CLINICAL COURSE: Suvival into adulthood has been documented.

CYTOGENETICS: Reported patients are the result of a de novo defect.

REFERENCES

Jalal SM, Macias VR, Roop H, Morgan F, King P. 1989. Two rare cases of 6p partial deletion. *Clin. Genet.* 36:196–199.

Kormann-Bortolotto MH, Farah LM, Soares D, Corbani M, Muller R, Adell AC. 1990. Terminal deletion 6p23: a case report. *Am. J. Med. Genet.* 37:475–477.

Palmer CG, Bader P, Slovak ML, Comings DE, Pettenati MJ. 1991. Partial deletion of chromosome 6p: delineation of the syndrome. *Am. J. Med. Genet.* 39:155–160.

Plaja A, Vidal R, Soriano D, Bou X, Vendrell T, Mediano C, Pueyo JM, Labrana X, Sarret E. 1994. Terminal deletion of 6p: report of a new case. *Ann. Genet.* 37:196–199.

Zurcher VL, Golden WL, Zinn AB. 1990. Distal deletion of the short arm of chromosome 6. *Am. J. Med. Genet.* 35:261–265.

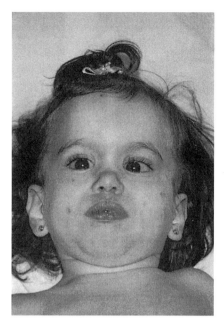
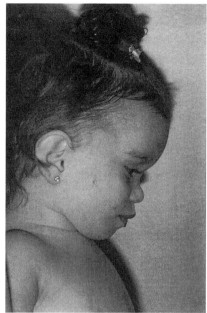

Patient at 3 years and 6 months. Note bulging forehead, prominent philtrum, low nasal bridge, strabismus, epicanthal folds, and low-set ears with prominence of antihelices. (From Plaja et al., 1994. *Ann. Genet.* 37:196–199. Reprinted with permission from Expansion Scientifique Francaise.)

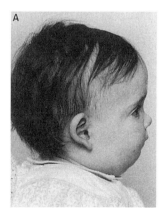
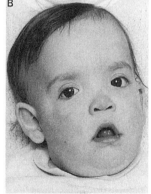

Patient at 1 year. Note mild biparietal narrowing, telecanthus, short, downward-slanting palpebral fissures, mild epicanthal folds, ears with cupping and malformed antihelices, broad, flat nasal bridge, short anteverted nose, tented upper lip, micrognathia, and short neck. (From Zurcher et al., 1990. *Am. J. Med. Genet.* 35:261–265. Copyright © 1990 John Wiley & Sons, Inc. Reprinted by permission of Wiley-Liss, Inc.)

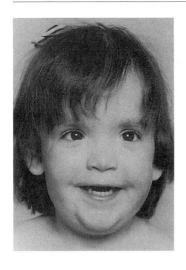

Patient at 2 years and 3 months. Note mild synophrys and flat philtrum. (From Zurcher et al., 1990. *Am. J. Med. Genet.* 35:261–265. Copyright © 1990 John Wiley & Sons, Inc. Reprinted by permission of Wiley-Liss, Inc.)

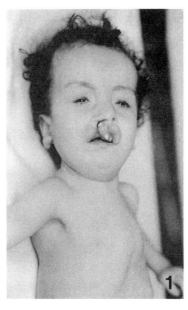

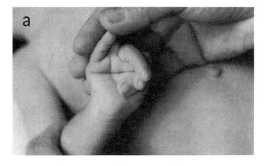

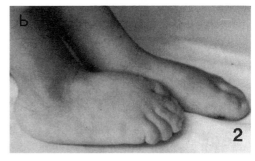

Patient at 2 years and 2 months. Note broad forehead, frontal bossing, downward-slanting palpebral fissures, telecanthus, microphthalmia, dysplastic, low-set ears, and unilateral cleft lip. (From Kormann-Bortolotto et al., 1990. *Am. J. Med. Genet.* 37:475–477. Copyright © 1990 John Wiley & Sons, Inc. Reprinted by permission of Wiley-Liss, Inc.)

Note simian crease, prominent heels, and partial syndactyly. (From Kormann-Bortolotto et al., 1990. *Am. J. Med. Genet.* 37:475–477. Copyright © 1990 John Wiley & Sons, Inc. Reprinted by permission of Wiley-Liss, Inc.)

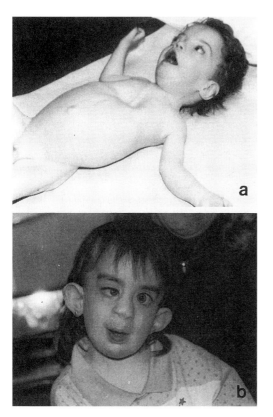
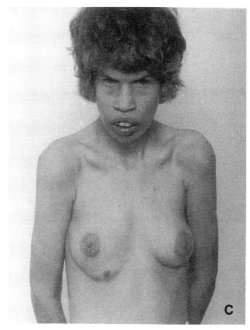

Patient at 13.5 months (a). Note pectus excavatum and unusual facies. Note right internal strabismus, flat, broad nasal bridge, large protruding ears, and repaired bilateral cleft lip (b). Note recessed eyes, micrognathia, and accessory nipple (c). (From Palmer et al., 1991. *Am. J. Med. Genet.* 39:155–160. Copyright © 1991 John Wiley & Sons, Inc. Reprinted by permission of Wiley-Liss, Inc.)

CHROMOSOME 6q PARTIAL TRISOMY

A definite syndrome is associated with the partial duplication of the long arm of chromosome 6.

MAIN FEATURES: Profound mental retardation, carp-shaped mouth, abnormally shaped skull, prominent forehead

ABNORMALITIES

Growth: Pre- and postnatal growth retardation

Performance: Profound mental retardation, feeding problems, psychomotor retardation

Eyes: Hypertelorism, abnormally shaped eyes

Craniofacies: Prominent forehead, short/webbed neck, acrocephaly, microcephaly, brachycephaly, turricephaly, telecanthus, low-set/rotated ears, broad nasal bridge, short philtrum, micrognathia, carp-shaped mouth, high-arched palate, downward-slanting palpebral fissures

Other: Hand and foot anomalies, joint contractures, bilateral simian crease, heart defects/murmur, genital anomalies

CLINICAL COURSE: Half of the babies reported were stillborn or died soon after birth. When there were less severe birth defects, survival was reported up to 22 years.

CYTOGENETICS: Patients may arise from a de novo defect or a parental chromosomal rearrangement.

REFERENCES

Giardino D, Rizzi N, Briscioli V, Bettio D. 1994. A de novo 6q11–q15 duplication investigated by chromosome painting. *Clin. Genet.* 46:377–379.

Henegariu O, Heerema NA, Vance GH. 1997. Mild "duplication 6q syndrome": a case with partial trisomy (6)(q23.3q25.3). *Am. J. Med. Genet.* 68:450–454.

Neu RL, Gallien JU, Steinberg-Warren N, Wynn RJ, Bannerman RM. 1981. An infant with trisomy 6q21 leads to 6qter. *Ann. Genet.* 24:167–179.

Pivnick EK, Qumsiyeh MB, Tharapel AT, Summitt JB, Wilroy RS. 1990. Partial duplication of the long arm of chromosome 6: a clinically recognisable syndrome. *J. Med. Genet.* 27:523–526.

Roland B, Lowry RB, Cox DM, Ferreira P, Lin CC. 1993. Familial complex chromosomal rearrangement resulting in duplication/deletion of 6q14 to 6q16. *Clin. Genet.* 43:117–121.

Taysi K, Chao WT, Monaghan N, Monaco MP. 1983. Trisomy 6q22 leads to 6qter due to maternal 6;21 translocation. Case report review of the literature. *Ann. Genet.* 26:243–246.

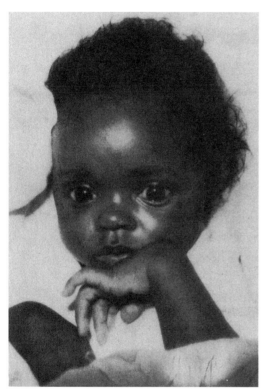
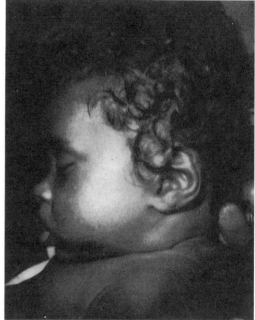

Patient at age 2 months. Note prominent occiput, prominent forehead, horizontal almond-shaped palpebral fissures, infraorbital creases, hypertelorism, broad, depressed nasal bridge, short philtrum, midface hypoplasia, carp-shaped mouth, and short neck. (From Henegariu et al., 1997. *Am. J. Med. Genet.* 68:450–454. Copyright © 1997 John Wiley & Sons, Inc. Reprinted by permission of Wiley-Liss, Inc.)

CHROMOSOME 6q PARTIAL MONOSOMY

Patients with deletions of 6q are relatively rare. To date, there has not been a specific syndrome associated with this defect, although there are characteristic features of monosomy 6q1. Some of the expected features of monosomy 6q1 include short neck, round face, minor facial anomalies, growth retardation, mental retardation, and hypotonia. Partial deletions of 6q occur in varying regions from patient to patient, which is likely to contribute to the phenotypic variation.

MAIN FEATURES: Large, malformed, low-set ears, hypotonia, growth retardation, and mental retardation.

ABNORMALITIES

Growth: Growth retardation

Performance: Mental retardation and hypotonia

Craniofacies: Abnormal head shape, large, malformed, low-set ears, abnormal palepebral fissures, hypertelorism, abnormal mouth, micrognathia, abnormal philtrum, and short neck

Genitourinary: Genital abnormalities

Limbs: Abnormal hands and feet

Other: Highly arched palate, strabismus, nystagmus, umbilical hernia, short stature, and hyperextensible skin.

OCCASIONAL ABNORMALITIES: Blue sclera, microcephaly, bulbous nose, epicanthal folds, retrognathia, abnormal palmar creases, low hairline, sparse hair, poor feeding, speech delay, psychomotor retardation, hemangioma, widely spaced nipples, and anteriorly displaced anus

CLINICAL COURSE: Death in infancy is not uncommon.

CYTOGENETICS: Most patients result from parental chromosomal rearrangements, but de novo defects have been reported.

REFERENCES

Gershoni-Baruch R, Mandel H, Bar El H, Bar-Nizan N, Borochowitz Z, Dar H. 1996. Interstitial deletion (6)q13q15. *Am. J. Med. Genet.* 62:345–347.

Horigome H, Takano T, Hirano T, Kajima T, Ohtani S. 1991. Interstitial deletion of the long arm of chromosome 6 associated with absent pulmonary valve. *Am. J. Med. Genet.* 38:608–611.

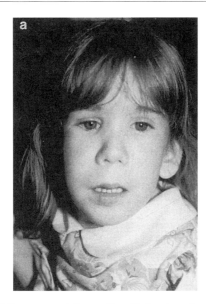
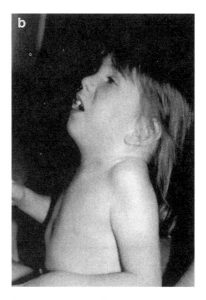

Patient at 3 years and 3 months. Note abundant light-colored scalp hair, large ears, smooth philtrum, mild retrognathia, and short neck with webbing. (From Romie et al., 1996. *Am. J. Med. Genet.* 62:105–108. Copyright © 1996 John Wiley & Sons, Inc. Reprinted by permission of Wiley-Liss, Inc.)

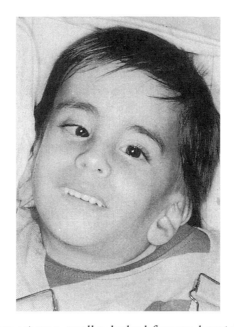

Patient at 2 years. Note deep-set eyes, small palpebral fissures, hypotelorism, strabismus, upward-slanting palpebral fissures, mild synophrys, large, posteriorly rotated, low-set ears with large pinnae, low frontal hairline, slender nose with small anteverted nostrils, flat maxillae, and micrognathia. (From Gershoni-Baruch et al., 1996. *Am. J. Med. Genet.* 62:345–347. Copyright © 1996 John Wiley & Sons, Inc. Reprinted by permission of Wiley-Liss, Inc.)

Lonardo F, Colantuoni M, Festa B, Gentile G, Guerritore G, Perone L, Santulli B, Ventruto V. 1988. A malformed girl with a de novo proximal 6q deletion. *Ann. Genet.* 31:57–59.

Pandya A, Braverman N, Pyeritz RE, Ying KL, Kline AD, Falk RE. 1995. Interstitial deletion of the long arm of chromosome 6 associated with unusual limb anomalies: report of two new patients and review of the literature. *Am. J. Med. Genet.* 59:38–43.

Romie SS, Hartsfield JK Jr, Sutcliffe MJ, Dumont DP, Kousseff BG. 1996. Monosomy 6q1: syndrome delineation. *Am. J. Med. Genet.* 62:105–108.

Villa A, Urioste M, Bofarull JM, Martinez-Frias ML. 1995. De novo interstitial deletion q16.2q21 on chromosome 6. *Am. J. Med. Genet.* 55:379–383.

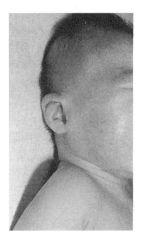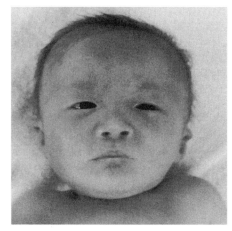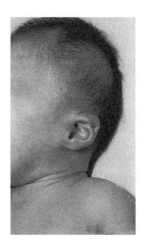

Patient at 1 month. Note facial flattening, borderline hypertelorism, low-set, small malformed ears, flat nasal bridge, bulbous nose, micrognathia, and thin vermillion border. (From Horigome et al., 1991. *Am. J. Med. Genet.* 38:608–611. Copyright © 1991 John Wiley & Sons, Inc. Reprinted by permission of Wiley-Liss, Inc.)

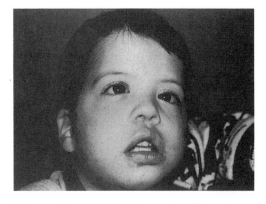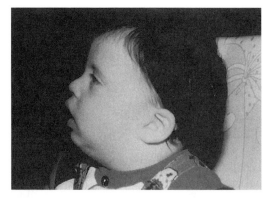

Patient at 1 year and 11 months. Note almond-shaped eyes, bilateral epicanthus and strabismus, downward-slanting palpebral fissures, bulbous nose, round cheeks, apparently low-set and posteriorly angulated ears, marked philtrum, fish mouth, everted lower lip, and mild retrognathia. (From Villa et al., 1995. *Am. J. Med. Genet.* 55:379–383. Copyright © 1995 John Wiley & Sons, Inc. Reprinted by permission of Wiley-Liss, Inc.)

RING CHROMOSOME 6

Many of the features of ring 6 are similar to those in del(6)(pter → q25:). Variability, however, does exist between ring 6 and del(6)(pter → q25:) individuals, most likely because of the varying size of the ring formation.

MAIN FEATURES: Microcephaly, micrognathia, eye and ear abnormalities, growth retardation

ABNORMALITIES

Growth: Low birth weight, growth retardation

Performance: Mental retardation, developmental delay, psychomotor retardation

Craniofacies: Microcephaly, hydrocephalus, low-set, malformed ears, high-arched palate, micrognathia, short neck, hypertelorism, epicanthal folds, flat, broad nasal bridge

Other: Central nervous system (CNS) malformations, talipes equinovalgus

OCCASIONAL ABNORMALITIES: Respiratory distress, seizures, congenital heart defects, hemivertebrae, bone age retardation

CLINICAL COURSE: Life span has been found to be 5 days to adulthood, depending on the severity of the birth defects present.

CYTOGENETICS: Usually sporadic

REFERENCES

Chitayat D, Hahm SY, Iqbal MA, Nitowsky HM. 1987. Ring chromosome 6: report of a patient and literature review. *Am. J. Med. Genet.* 26:145–151.

Fryns JP, Kleczkowska A, van den Berghe H. 1990. Ring chromosome 6: twenty years follow-up. *Ann. Genet.* 33:179.

Kini KR, Van Dyke DL, Weiss L, Logan MS. 1979. Ring chromosome 6: case report and review of literature. *Hum. Genet.* 50:145–149.

Paz-y-Mino C, Benitez J, Ayuso C, Sanchez-Cascos A. 1990. Ring chromosome 6: clinical and cytogenetic behaviour. *Am. J. Med. Genet.* 35:481–483.

Peeden JN, Scarbrough P, Taysi K, Wilroy RS, Finley S, Luthardt F, Martens P, Howard-Peebles PN. 1983. Ring chromosome 6: variability in phenotypic expression. *Am. J. Med. Genet.* 16:563–573.

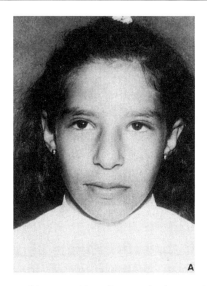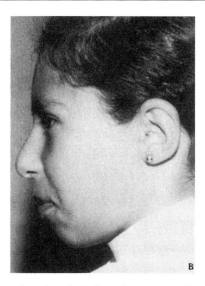

Patient at age 10 years. Note hypertelorism, epicanthus, low hair line, low-set, malformed ears, and micrognathia. (From Paz-y-Miño et al., 1990. *Am. J. Med. Genet.* 35:481–483. Copyright © 1990 John Wiley & Sons, Inc. Reprinted by permission of Wiley-Liss, Inc.)

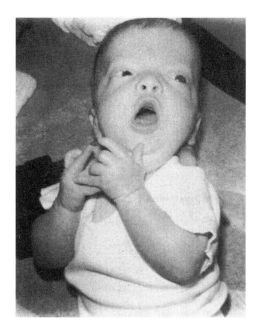

Patient at age 3 months. Note microcephaly, downward-slanting palpebral fissures, hypertelorism, small, low-set, posteriorly angulated ears, small, pointed nose, anteverted nares, microstomia, and short neck. (From Chitayat et al., 1987. *Am. J. Med. Genet.* 26:145–151. Copyright © 1987 John Wiley & Sons, Inc. Reprinted by permission of Wiley-Liss, Inc.)

Sele B, Joannard A, Jalbert P, Boucharlat J. 1977. [Ring 6-chromosome: a nonspecific clinical picture]. *Ann. Genet.* 20:232–236.

Walker ME, Lynch-Salamon DA, Milatovich A, Saal HM. 1996. Prenatal diagnosis of ring chromosome 6 in a fetus with hydrocephalus. *Prenat. Diagn.* 16:857–861.

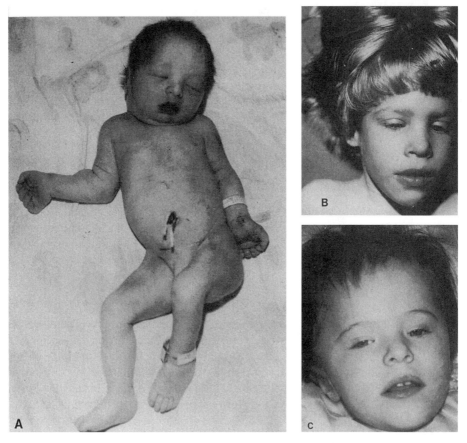

Patient at age 3 days (A), 6 years (B), and 1 year and 6 months (C). Note round face, flat supraorbital ridges, downward-slanting palpebral fissures, low-set ears, prominent eyes, wide, prominent nasal bridge contiguous with the forehead, cupid's bow upper lip, and micrognathia. (From Peeden et al., 1983. *Am. J. Med. Genet.* 16:563–573. Copyright © 1983 John Wiley & Sons, Inc. Reprinted by permission of Wiley-Liss, Inc.)

CHROMOSOME 7p PARTIAL TRISOMY

Although patients with partial trisomy for 7p are relatively rare, a characteristic phenotype has been identified. A majority of these patients will present with head and skull abnormalities, including wide, large fontanelles and a high forehead. Reported patients usually result from de novo defects.

MAIN FEATURES: Head and skull abnormalities, low-set ears, and mental retardation

ABNORMALITIES

Performance: Developmental delay, speech delay, mental retardation, hypotonia, failure to thrive

Craniofacies: Head and skull abnormalities, wide, large fontanelle, high forehead, malformed, low-set ears, downward-slanting palpebral fissures, beaked nose

Limbs: Abnormal hands and feet with abnormal fingers and toes

Other: Abnormal chest, patent ductus arteriosus, highly arched palate

OCCASIONAL ABNORMALITIES: Imperforate anus, cryptorchidism, hypertelorism, abnormal palmar creases, heart murmur

CLINICAL COURSE: Death in infancy is not uncommon.

CYTOGENETICS: In almost all cases, the defects are de novo, but familial chromosomal rearrangements have been found.

REFERENCES

Debiec-Rychter M, Overhauser J, Kaluzewski B, Jakubowski L, Truszczak B, Wilson W, Skorski M, Jackson L. 1990. De novo direct tandem duplication of the short arm of chromosome 7(p21.1-p14.2). *Am. J. Med. Genet.* 36:316–320.

Franz HB, Schliephacke M, Niemann G, Mielke G, Backsch C. 1996. De novo direct tandem duplication of a small segment of the short arm of chromosome 7(p21.22 → 22.1). *Clin. Genet.* 50:426–429.

Pallotta R, Dalpra L, Fusilli P, Zuffardi O. 1996. Further delineation of 7p trisomy. Case report and review of literature. *Ann. Genet.* 39:152–158.

Park JP, McDermet MK, Moeschler JB, Wurster-Hill DH. 1993. A case of de novo translocation 7; 10 and the duplication 7p, deletion 10p phenotype. *Ann. Genet.* 36:217–220.

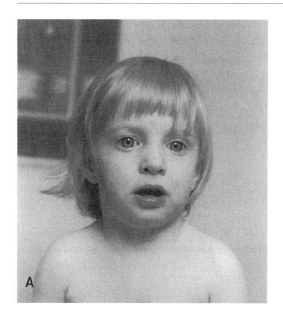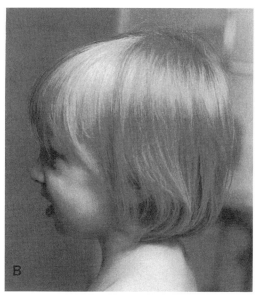

Patient at 1 year and 8 months. Note normal appearance. (From Schafer et al., 1995. *Am. J. Med. Genet.* 56:184–187. Copyright © 1995 John Wiley & Sons, Inc. Reprinted by permission of Wiley-Liss, Inc.)

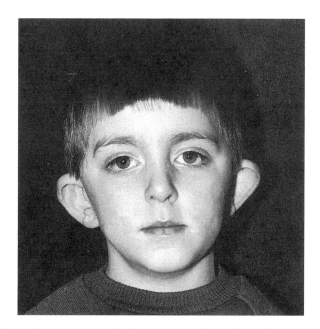

Patient at 6 years. Note floppy, apparently low-set ears, hypoplastic helices, small mandible, downward-slanting palpebral fissures, and ptosis. (From Debiec-Rychter et al., 1990. *Am. J. Med. Genet.* 36:316–320. Copyright © 1990 John Wiley & Sons, Inc. Reprinted by permission of Wiley-Liss, Inc.)

Redha MA, Krishna Murthy DS, al-Awadi SA, al-Sulaiman IS, Sabry MA, el-Bahey SA, Farag TI. 1996. De novo direct duplication 7p(p11.2 → pter) in an Arab child with MCA/MR syndrome: trisomy 7p a dilineated syndrome? *Ann. Genet.* 39:5–9.

Reish O, Berry SA, Dewald G, King RA. 1996. Duplication of 7p: further delineation of the phenotype and restriction of the critical region to the distal part of the short arm. *Am J. Med. Genet.* 61:21–25.

Schaefer GB, Novak K, Steele D, Buehler B, Smith S, Zaleski D, Pickering D, Nelson M, Sanger W. 1995. Familial inverted duplication 7p. *Am. J. Med. Genet.* 56:184–187.

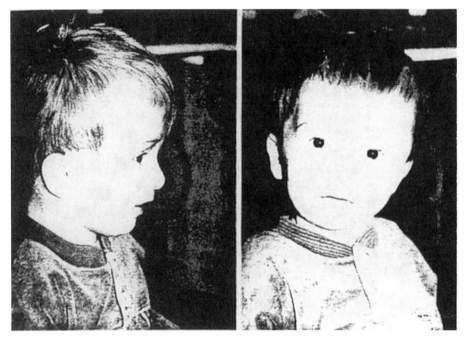

Patient at 1 year and 8 months. Note high forehead, hypertelorism, slightly downward-slanting palpebral fissures, and low-set ears. (From Franz et al., 1996. *Clin. Genet.* 50:426–429. Copyright © 1996 Munksgaard International Publishers Ltd., Copenhagen, Denmark, with permission.)

CHROMOSOME 7p PARTIAL MONOSOMY

Partial monosomy for 7p has been noted to produce enormous phenotypic variability. This variability most likely occurs due to patient differences in the size and location of the deletion. This region of the chromosome is large; therefore it contains numerous genes that, when disrupted or deleted, will result in some of the features previously described in monosomy 7p. Further delineation of 7p will clarify associations between features and their corresponding chromosomal band. Greig syndrome, which includes postaxial polydactyly and facial dysmorphism, has been localized to 7p13.

MAIN FEATURES: Craniosynostosis, epicanthal folds, and growth retardation

ABNORMALITIES

Growth: Growth retardation

Performance: Developmental delay and mental retardation

Craniofacies: Craniosynostosis, abnormal head shape, malformed ears, broad, flat nasal bridge, high-arched palate, downward-slanting palpebral fissures, and epicanthal folds

Genitourinary: Urogenital abnormalities

Limbs: Abnormal hands and feet with abnormal fingers and toes

Other: Pectus excavatum and umbilical hernia

OCCASIONAL ABNORMALITIES: Low-set ears, hypertelorism, syndactyly, cardiac defects, failure to thrive, low hairline, speech delay, and seizures

CLINICAL COURSE: Death in infancy is not uncommon, but survival into adulthood has been documented.

CYTOGENETICS: In almost all cases the defects are de novo.

REFERENCES

Aughton DJ, Cassidy SB, Whiteman DA, Delach JA, Guttmacher AE. 1991. Chromosome 7p− syndrome: craniosynostosis with preservation of region 7p2. *Am. J. Med. Genet.* 40:440–443.

Grebe TA, Stevens MA, Byrne-Essif K, Cassidy SB. 1992. 7p deletion syndrome: an adult with mild manifestations. *Am. J. Med. Genet.* 44:18–23.

Kikkawa K, Narahara K, Tsuji K, Kubo T, Yokoyama Y, Seino Y. 1993. Is loss of band 7p21 really critical for manifestation of craniosynostosis in 7p-? *Am. J. Med. Genet.* 45:108–110.

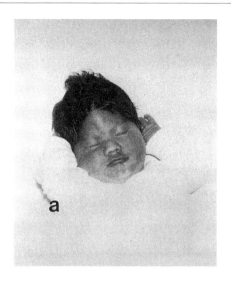

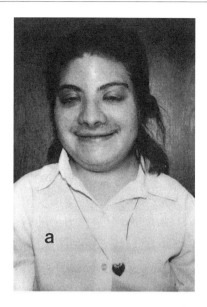

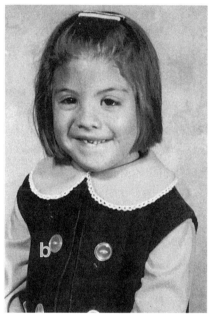

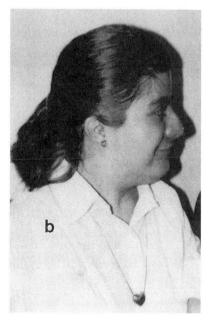

Patient at birth and 3 years. Note prow-shaped forehead and ptosis of the left eyelid. (From Grebe et al., 1992. *Am. J. Med. Genet.* 44:18–23. Copyright © 1992 John Wiley & Sons, Inc. Reprinted by permission of Wiley-Liss, Inc.)

Patient at 24 years. Note short forehead, low hairline, prominent glabella, hypertelorism, telecanthus, short, downward-slanting palpebral fissures, epicanthal folds, large nose, broad, prominent nasal bridge, short, poorly grooved philtrum, short, wide mouth, short ears, and short neck. (From Grebe et al., 1992. *Am. J. Med. Genet.* 44:18–23. Copyright © 1992 John Wiley & Sons, Inc. Reprinted by permission of Wiley-Liss, Inc.)

Pettigrew AL, Greenberg F, Caskey CT, Ledbetter DH. 1991. Greig syndrome associated with an interstitial deletion of 7p: confirmation of the localization of Greig syndrome to 7p13. *Hum. Genet.* 87:452–456.

Roberts SH, Hughes HE, Davies SJ, Meredith AL. 1991. Bilateral split hand and split foot malformation in a boy with a de novo interstitial deletion of 7q21.3. *J. Med. Genet.* 28:479–481.

Wang C, Maynard S, Glover TW, Biesecker LG. 1993. Mild phenotypic manifestation of a 7p15.3p21.2 deletion. *J. Med. Genet.* 30:610–612.

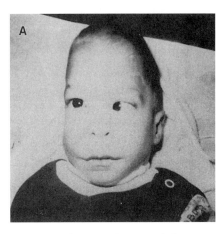
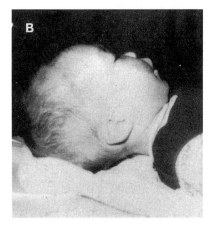

Patient at 1 year and 6 months. Note left esotropia, bilateral epicanthal folds, broad, flat nasal bridge, short, upturned nose, and long, wide philtrum. (From Aughton et al., 1991. *Am. J. Med. Genet.* 40:440–443. Copyright © 1991 John Wiley & Sons, Inc. Reprinted by permission of Wiley-Liss, Inc.)

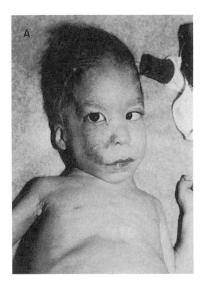
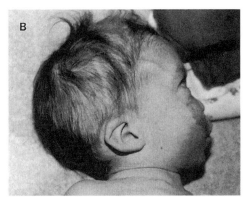

Patient at 2 years and 7 months. Note similar findings as at 1 year and 6 months. (From Aughton et al., 1991. *Am. J. Med. Genet.* 40:440–443. Copyright © 1991 John Wiley & Sons, Inc. Reprinted by permission of Wiley-Liss, Inc.)

CHROMOSOME 7q PARTIAL TRISOMY

Patients with partial trisomy 7q are rare. A characteristic phenotype has been described for individuals with this defect. Expected findings include mental retardation, hypotonia, skeletal defects, and low-set, malformed ears. Patients often result from familial chromosomal rearrangements; although de novo defects have been documented as well.

MAIN FEATURES: Mental retardation, hypotonia, and skeletal abnormalities

ABNORMALITIES

Performance: Developmental delay, mental retardation, and hypotonia

Craniofacies: Abnormal skull shape, macrocephaly, frontal bossing, malformed, low-set ears, downward-slanting palpebral fissures, abnormal nose, depressed nasal bridge, and epicanthal folds

Limbs: Abnormal hands and feet with abnormal fingers and toes, clinodactyly, and single palmar crease

Other: Skeletal anomalies

OCCASIONAL ABNORMALITIES: Short, webbed neck, large fontanelle, enlarged ventricles of brain, hypertelorism, high-arched palate, microretrognathia, strabismus, cardiac defects, kyphoscoliosis, and hip dislocation

CLINICAL COURSE: Survival into childhood has been documented.

CYTOGENETICS: Both familial chromosomal rearrangements and de novo defects have been documented.

REFERENCES

Bartsch O, Kalbe U, Ngo TK, Lettau R, Schwinger E. 1990. Clinical diagnosis of partial duplication 7q. *Am. J. Med. Genet.* 37:254–257.

Haslam JS, Norman AM. 1992. De novo inverted duplication of chromosome 7q. *J. Med. Genet.* 29:837–838.

Romain DR, Cairney H, Stewart D, Columbano-Green LM, Garry M, Parslow MI, Parfitt R, Smythe RH, Chapman CJ. 1990. Three cases of partial trisomy 7q owing to rare structural rearrangements of chromosome 7. *J. Med. Genet.* 27:109–113.

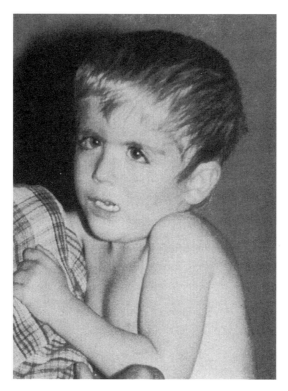

Patient at 3 years and 3 months. Note frontal bossing, slightly downward-sloping palpebral fissures, deep-set eyes, flared eyebrows, long eyelashes, and short nose. (From Stratton et al., 1993. *Am. J. Med. Genet.* 47:380–382. Copyright © 1993 John Wiley & Sons, Inc. Reprinted by permission of Wiley-Liss, Inc.)

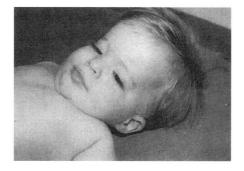

Patient at 9 months. Note macrocephaly, high forehead, frontal bossing, deep nasal bridge, epicanthal folds, downward-slanting palpebral fissures, low-set ears, slight microretrognathia, and short neck. (From Bartsch et al., 1990. *Am. J. Med. Genet.* 37:254–257. Copyright © 1990 John Wiley & Sons, Inc. Reprinted by permission of Wiley-Liss, Inc.)

Stetten G, Charity LL, Kasch LM, Scott AF, Berman CL, Pressman E, Blakemore KJ. 1997. A paternally derived inverted duplication of 7q with evidence of a telomeric deletion. *Am. J. Med. Genet.* 68:76–81.

Stratton RF, DuPont BR, Mattern VL, Schelonka RL, Moore CM. 1993. Interstitial duplication of 7(q22 → q34). *Am. J. Med. Genet.* 47:380–382.

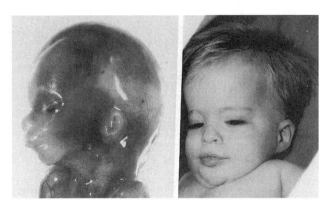

Note that the faces of the boy and the fetus have similar features. (From Bartsch et al., 1990. *Am. J. Med. Genet.* 37:254–257. Copyright © 1990 John Wiley & Sons, Inc. Reprinted by permission of Wiley-Liss, Inc.)

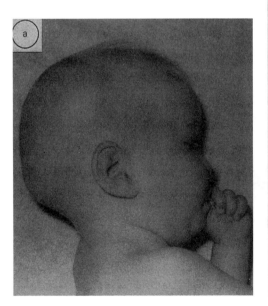
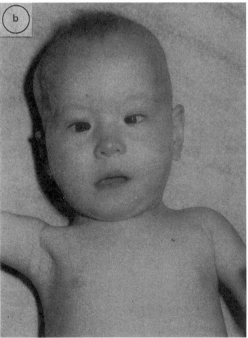

Note frontal bossing, depressed nasal bridge, epicanthal folds, and fixed, convergent squint. (From Romain et al., 1990. *J. Med. Genet.* 27:109–113. Reprinted with permission from BMJ Publishing Group.)

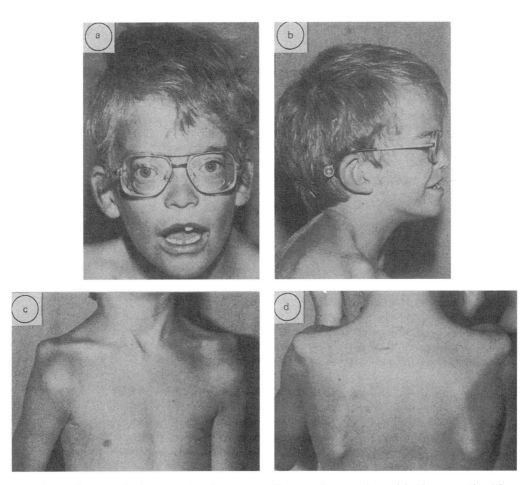

Note glasses for myopia, low-set, simple ears, small nose, depressed nasal bridge, mouth with a thin upper lip, abnormal teeth, congenital bilateral anterior dislocation of the shoulders, and kyphoscoliosis. (From Romain et al., 1990. *J. Med. Genet.* 27:109–113. Reprinted with permission from BMJ Publishing Group.)

CHROMOSOME 7q PARTIAL MONOSOMY

Patients with monosomy 7q are rare but often are found to present with similar features. Consistently noted features include developmental delay, growth retardation, unusual facial appearance, and abnormal electroencephalogram. Microdeletions of 7q11.23 are well known to result in Williams syndrome.

MAIN FEATURES: Mental retardation, unusual facial appearance, abnormal electroencephalogram

ABNORMALITIES

Growth: Growth retardation

Performance: Developmental delay, mental retardation, poor feeding

Craniofacies: Abnormal skull shape, microcephaly, malformed, low-set ears, abnormal nose, broad nasal bridge, hypertelorism, micrognathia, abnormal mouth, eye abnormalities

Genitourinary: Genital abnormalities in males

Limbs: Abnormal hands and feet, ectrodactyly, clinodactyly, abnormal palmar creases

Other: Inguinal hernia, cardiac defects, seizures, abnormal electroencephalogram

OCCASIONAL ABNORMALITIES: Hearing loss, cleft lip and/or palate, hypotonia, joint contractures/scoliosis, holoprosencephaly

CLINICAL COURSE: Death in infancy has been documented.

CYTOGENETICS: In almost all cases, the defects are de novo, but familial chromosomal rearrangements have been found.

REFERENCES

Bogart MH, Cunniff C, Bradshaw C, Jones KL, Jones OW. 1990. Terminal deletions of the long arm of chromosome 7: five new cases. *Am. J. Med. Genet.* 36:53–55.

Brondum-Nielsen K, Beck B, Gyftodimou J, Horlyk H, Liljenberg U, Petersen MB, Pedersen W, Petersen MB, Sand A, Skovby F, Stafanger G, Zetterqvist P, Tommerup N. 1997. Investigation of deletions at 7q11.23 in 44 patients referred for Williams-Beuren syndrome, using FISH and four DNA polymorphisms. *Hum. Genet.* 99:56–61.

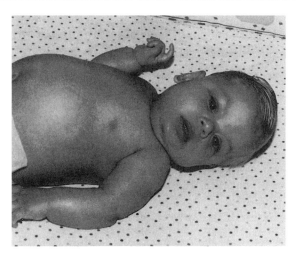

Patient at 1 year and 2 months. Note mild ptosis of the left eye, depressed nasal root, wide nasal bridge, upturned nose, and anteverted nares. (From Gillar et al., 1992. *Am. J. Med. Genet.* 44:138–141. Copyright © 1992 John Wiley & Sons, Inc. Reprinted by permission of Wiley-Liss, Inc.)

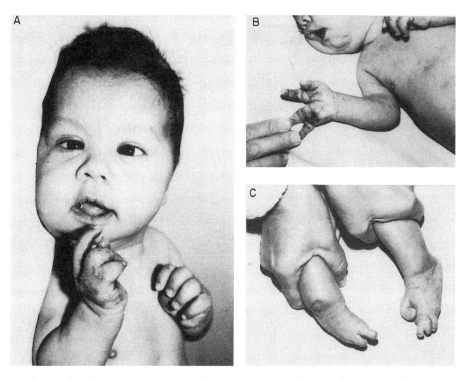

Patient at 3 months. Note convergent strabismus, anteverted nares, long upper lip, micrognathia, malformed ears, ectrodactyly of the right hand, and ectrodactyly of both feet. (From Tajara et al., 1989. *Am. J. Med. Genet.* 32:192–194. Copyright © 1989 John Wiley & Sons, Inc. Reprinted by permission of Wiley-Liss, Inc.)

D'Alessandro E, Ligas C, Lo Re ML, Marcanio MP, Gentile T, Del Porto G. 1994. Partial monosomy of 7q32 in a case of de novo rcp(7;15)(q32;q15). *J. Med. Genet.* 31:413–415.

Gillar PJ, Kaye CI, Ryan SG, Moore CM. 1992. Proximal 7q interstitial deletion in a severely mentally retarded and mildly abnormal infant. *Am. J. Med. Genet.* 44:138–141.

Morey MA, Higgins RR. 1990. Ectro-amelia syndrome associated with an interstitial deletion of 7q. *Am. J. Med. Genet.* 35:95–99.

Tajara EH, Varella-Garcia M, Gusson AC. 1989. Interstitial long-arm deletion of chromosome 7 and ectrodactyly. *Am. J. Med. Genet.* 32:192–194.

Tsukamoto H, Inui K, Taniike M, Kamiyama K, Hori M, Sumi K, Okada S. 1993. Different clinical features in monozygotic twins: a case of 7q−syndrome. *Clin. Genet.* 43:139–142.

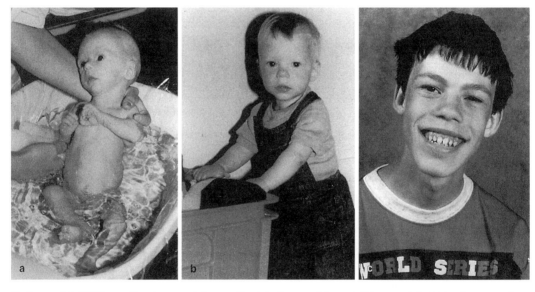

Patient with Williams Syndrome at 2 months (a), 1 year (b), and 15 years (c). Note downward-slanting palpebral fissures, epicanthal folds, periorbital fullness, full cheeks, upturned nose, long philtrum, wide mouth, and widely spaced teeth. (From Brandum-Nielsen et al., 1997. *Hum. Genet.* 99:56–61. Copyright © 1997 Springer-Verlag. Reprinted with permission.)

RING CHROMOSOME 7

Patients presenting with ring chromosome 7 are extremely rare. The associated features are variable, although most patients exhibit growth retardation, microcephaly, and dermatological abnormalities. It has been suggested that the phenotypic variation may result from differences in the size of the chromosomal deletion or ring chromosome instability resulting in mosaicism.

MAIN FEATURES: Growth retardation, microcephaly, and dermatological abnormalities

ABNORMALITIES

Growth: Low birth weight, growth retardation, short stature

Performance: Develpmental delay, mental retardation

Craniofacies: Microcephaly, abnormally spaced eyes

Skin: Dermatological findings including cafe-au-lait spot, pigmented nevi, hemangioma, nevi flammeus

Genitourinary: Small penis

Other: Bone abnormalities, widely spaced nipples

OCCASIONAL ABNORMALITIES: Small ears, cleft lip, cleft palate, holoprosencephaly

CLINICAL COURSE: Death in infancy is not uncommon, but survival to adulthood has been documented.

CYTOGENETICS: Reported patients are the result of a de novo defect.

REFERENCES

DeLozier CD, Theintz G, Sizonenko P, Engel E. 1982. A fourth case of ring chromosome 7. *Clin. Genet.* 22:90–98.

Koiffmann CP, Diament A, de Souza DH, Wajntal A. 1990. Ring chromosome 7 in a man with multiple congenital anomalies and mental retardation. *J. Med. Genet.* 27:462–464.

Sawyer JR, Lukacs JL, Hassed SJ, Arnold GL, Mitchell HF, Muenke M. 1996. Sub-band deletion of 7q36.3 in a patient with ring chromosome 7: association with holoprosencephaly. *Am. J. Med. Genet.* 65:113–116.

Tsukamoto H, Sakai N, Taniike M, Nakatsukasa M, Yoshiwara W, Sakamoto H, Fujimura H, Inui K, Okada S. 1993. Case of ring chromosome 7: the first report of neuropathological findings. *Am. J. Med. Genet.* 46:632–635.

Wahlstrom J, Bjarnason R, Rosdahl I, Albertsson-Wikland K. 1996. Boy with a ring 7 chromosome: a case report with special reference to dermatological findings. *Acta Paediatr.* 85:1256–1260.

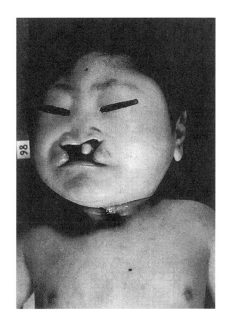

Note hypertelorism, upward-slanting palpebral fissures, broad nasal root, defect of nasal tip, bilateral cleft lip, and small, low-set ears. (From Tsukamoto et al., 1993. *Am. J. Med. Genet.* 46:632–635. Copyright © 1993 John Wiley & Sons, Inc. Reprinted by permission of Wiley-Liss, Inc.)

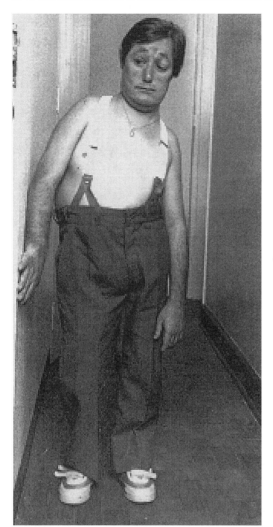

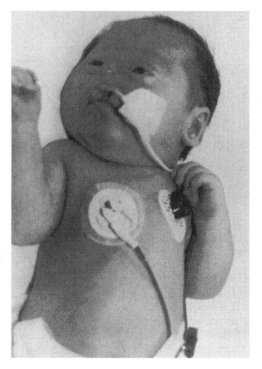

Note hypotelorism, with proptosis, flat proboscis with a single nostril, and midline cleft lip. (From Sawyer et al., 1996. *Am. J. Med. Genet.* 65:113–116. Copyright © 1996 John Wiley & Sons, Inc. Reprinted by permission of Wiley-Liss, Inc.)

Patient at 39 years of age. Note ptosis of the right eyelid, hypotelorism, upward-slanting eyebrows, beaked nose, high-set ears, thin lips, long philtrum, malar hypoplasia, kyphoscoliosis, and pigmented nevi mainly on the back and abdomen. (From Koiffmann et al., 1990. *J. Med. Genet.* 27:462–464. Reprinted with permission from BMJ Publishing Group.)

CHROMOSOME 8p PARTIAL TRISOMY

Individuals with partial trisomy 8p present with some predictable features. In addition, it has been noted that facial features of affected individuals generally become more coarse in appearance as they age. Most cases of partial trisomy 8p are the result of parental chromosomal rearrangements.

MAIN FEATURES: Mental retardation, hypotonia, agenesis of the corpus callosum

ABNORMALITIES

Performance: Mental retardation, hypotonia

Brain: Agenesis of the corpus callosum, enlarged cerebral ventricles

Craniofacies: Prominent forehead, broad nasal bridge, anteverted nostrils, prominent nose, sagging cheeks, eversion of lower lip, large mouth, long philtrum, large ears, temporal baldness

Other: Orthopedic problems, highly arched palate

OCCASIONAL ABNORMALITIES: Scoliosis and/or kyphosis, micrognathia, eye anomalies, short neck, slender extremeties, long trunk, contractures of large joints, long fingers

CLINICAL COURSE: Death in infancy is uncommon.

CYTOGENETICS: Most cases are the result of a de novo defect.

REFERENCES

de Die-Smulders CE, Engelen JJ, Schrander-Stumpel CT, Govaerts LC, de Vries B, Vles JS, Wagemans A, Schijns-Fleuren S, Gillessen-Kaesbach G, Fryns JP. 1995. Inversion duplication of the short arm of chromosome 8: clinical data on seven patients and review of the literature. *Am. J. Med. Genet.* 59:369–374.

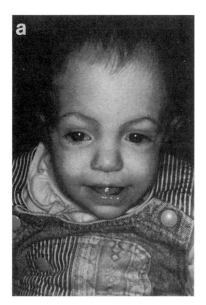
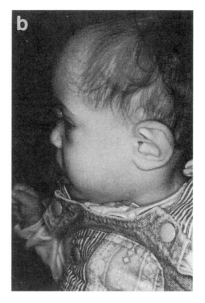

Note frontal bossing, bulbous nose, and large, simple ear. (From Guo et al., 1995. *Am. J. Med. Genet.* 58:230–236. Copyright © 1995 John Wiley & Sons, Inc. Reprinted by permission of Wiley-Liss, Inc.)

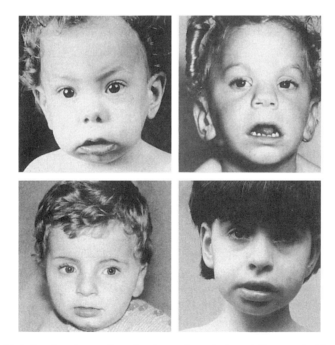

Note round face, high forehead, sagging cheeks, anteverted nostrils, everted lower lip, and curly hair. (From Die-Smulders et al., 1995. *Am. J. Med. Genet.* 59:369–374. Copyright © 1995 John Wiley & Sons, Inc. Reprinted by permission of Wiley-Liss, Inc.)

Digilio MC, Giannotti A, Floridia G, Uccellatore F, Mingarelli R, Danesino C, Dallapiccola B, Zuffardi O. 1994. Trisomy 8 syndrome owing to isodicentric 8p chromosomes: regional assignment of a presumptive gene involved in corpus callosum development. *J. Med. Genet.* 31:238–241.

Feldman GL, Weiss L, Phelan MC, Schroer RJ, Van Dyke DL. 1993. Inverted duplication of 8p: ten new patients and review of the literature. *Am. J. Med. Genet.* 47:482–486.

Guo WJ, Callif-Daley F, Zapata MC, Miller ME. 1995. Clinical and cytogenetic findings in seven cases of inverted duplication of 8p with evidence of a telomeric deletion using fluorescence in situ hybridization. *Am. J. Med. Genet.* 58:230–236.

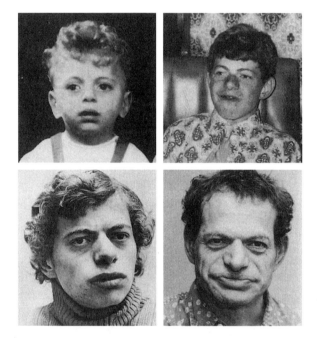

Note patient at different ages. Upper left as a toddler: high forehead, small nose with upturned nares, everted lower lip, large, slightly low-set ears, and curly hair with receding hairline in the temporal region. Upper right as an adolescent: coarsening of facial features. Lower left as a young adult: large nose, deep-set eyes, and large mouth with thick lips. Lower right, current appearance: coarse facial features, large nose and mouth, thick lips, everted lower lip, and large ears. (From Die-Smulders et al., 1995. *Am. J. Med. Genet.* 59:369–374. Copyright © 1995 John Wiley & Sons, Inc. Reprinted by permission of Wiley-Liss, Inc.)

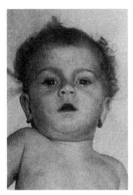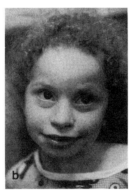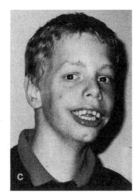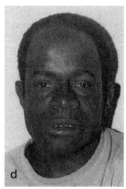

Patient 1 at age 1 year (a). Note broad forehead with frontal prominence, long philtrum, bow-shaped mouth with thin upper lip and large ears. Patient 2 age 7 (b). Note wide mouth with thin upper lip, prominent lower lip, and irregular teeth. Patient 3 at age 15 (c). Note prominent forehead, wide mouth with prominent lower lip, micrognathia, chin dimple, and dental anomalies. Patient 4 at age 30 (d). Note prominent forehead, wide mouth with widely spaced teeth and chin cleft. (From Feldman et al., 1993. *Am. J. Med. Genet.* 47:482–486. Copyright © 1993 John Wiley & Sons, Inc. Reprinted by permission of Wiley-Liss, Inc.)

CHROMOSOME 8p PARTIAL MONOSOMY

Partial monosomy 8p is a rare finding that often results in growth and mental retardation, congenital heart defects, and minor facial dysmorphism. In almost all cases, the defects are de novo, although, rarely, familial chromosomal rearrangements have been identified.

MAIN FEATURES: Growth and mental retardation, cardiac defects, dolichocephaly

ABNORMALITIES

Growth: Low birth weight, growth retardation

Performance: Developmental delay, mental retardation, speech delay

Craniofacies: Microcephaly, dolicocephaly, high, narrow forehead, malformed, low-set ears, abnormal palpebral fissures, epicanthal folds, short nose, flat nasal bridge, thin lips, abnormal chin

Genitourinary: Genital abnormalities

Other: Highly arched palate, micrognathia, short neck, broad chest, widely spaced nipples, cardiac defects

OCCASIONAL ABNORMALITIES: Hypertelorism, abnormal fingers, puffy hands

CLINICAL COURSE: Death in infancy has been documented.

CYTOGENETICS: Most cases are the result of a de novo defect, although familial chromosomal rearrangements have been documented.

REFERENCES

Blennow E, Brondum-Nielsen K. 1990. Partial monosomy 8p with minimal dysmorphic signs. *J. Med. Genet.* 27:327–329.

Marino B, Reale A, Giannotti A, Digilio MC, Dallapiccola B. 1992. Nonrandom association of atrioventricular canal and del (8p) syndrome. *Am. J. Med. Genet.* 42:424–427.

Morrison PJ, Jones J, Nevin NC. 1992. Interstitial deletion 8p21.3–p23.1 in a 6-year-old girl. *Am. J. Med. Genet.* 42:678–680.

Tsukahara M, Murano I, Aoki Y, Kajii T, Furukawa S. 1995. Interstitial deletion of 8p: report of two patients and review of the literature. *Clin. Genet.* 48:41–45.

Wu BL, Schneider GH, Sabatino DE, Bozovic LZ, Cao B, Korf BR. 1996. Distal 8p deletion (8)(p23.1): an easily missed chromosomal abnormality that may be associated with congenital heart defect and mental retardation. *Am. J. Med. Genet.* 62:77–83.

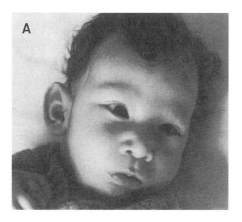

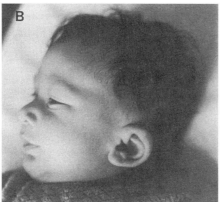

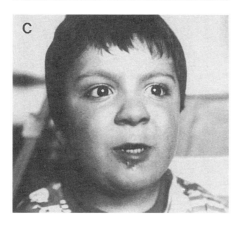

Patient at 2 months (A, B). Note high anterior hairline, prominent glabella, thin and sparse eyebrows, deep-set eyes, short and upward-slanted palpebral fissures, flat nasal bridge, broad-based nose, long upper lip, microstomia, anteverted lower lip, and micrognathia. Patient at 4 years (C). Note long, thin eyebrows, horizontal palpebral fissures, prominent nasal bridge, chubby cheeks, and a prominent lower lip with a horizontal groove on the chin. (From Marino et al., 1992. *Am. J. Med. Genet.* 42:424–427. Copyright © 1992 John Wiley & Sons, Inc. Reprinted by permission of Wiley-Liss, Inc.)

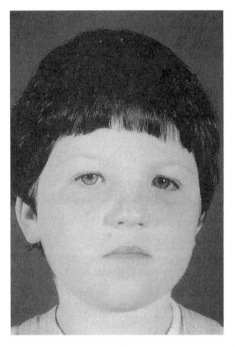 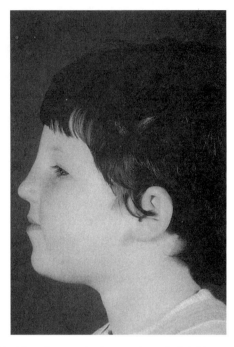

Patient at 6 years. Note high forehead, full nasal bridge, hypertelorism, epicanthal folds, small mouth, and low-set, posteriorly rotated ears with thickened helices. (From Morrison et al., 1992. *Am. J. Med. Genet.* 42:678–680. Copyright © 1992 John Wiley & Sons, Inc. Reprinted by permission of Wiley-Liss, Inc.)

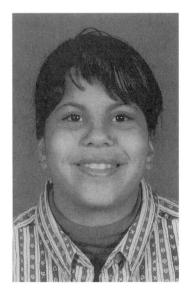 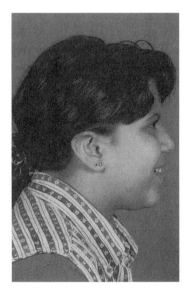

Patient at 9 years. Note almond-shaped, upward-slanting palpebral fissures, small head, and narrow forehead. (From Wu et al., 1996. *Am. J. Med. Genet.* 62:77–83. Copyright © 1996 John Wiley & Sons, Inc. Reprinted by permission of Wiley-Liss, Inc.)

CHROMOSOME 8q PARTIAL TRISOMY

Partial trisomy for chromosome 8q has been documented in numerous patients. The region of chromosome 8 that is duplicated varies between patients and appears to contribute to clinical variability. Several syndromes have been suggested, all of which are distinct from trisomy 8 mosaicism.

MAIN FEATURES: Mental retardation, thin upper lip, anteverted nares

ABNORMALITIES

Growth: Short stature

Performance: Mental retardation, poor feeding

Craniofacies: High, broad forehead, prominent frontal protuberances, abnormal pinnae and palpebral fissure slant, anteverted nares, thin upper lip, depressed nasal bridge, microretrognathia

Genitourinary: Genital anomalies including cryptorchidism and small penis and/or scrotum

Limbs: Abnormal toe posture, clinodactyly, abnormal palmar creases, distal axial triradius

Other: Cardiac defects and broad, short neck

OCCASIONAL ABNORMALITIES: Microcephaly, long philtrum, broad nasal root, large ears, abnormal eyebrows

CLINICAL COURSE: Death in infancy is uncommon.

CYTOGENETICS: Most cases are the result of a de novo defect, although familial chromosomal rearrangements have been reported.

REFERENCES

Donnenfeld AE, Coyne MD, Beauregard LJ. 1990. De novo inverted interstitial ("mirror") duplication of chromosome 8(q13 → q24.1) in a liveborn male. *Am. J. Med. Genet.* 35:529–531.

Sachs ES, van Waveren G. 1981. Phenotype of partial trisomy 8 (p21 leads to qter) in two unrelated patients with de novo translocation. *J. Med. Genet.* 18:204–208.

Stengel-Rutkowski S, Lohse K, Herzog C, Apacik C, Couturier J, Albert A, Belohradsky B. 1992. Partial trisomy 8q. Two case reports with maternal translocation and inverted insertion: phenotype analyses and reflections on the risk. *Clin. Genet.* 42:178–185.

Tupler R, Pagliano E, Barbierato L, Lanzi G, Maraschio P, Fazzi E. 1996. Mild phenotype associated with inv dup 8(q21.2 → q22.3) of maternal origin. *Am. J. Med. Genet.* 62:160–163.

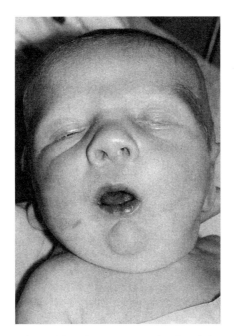

Patient at 7 days, note square-shaped head, prominent forehead, hypertelorism, wide nasal bridge, prominent upturned nose, low-set, posteriorly angulated ears, and micrognathia. (From Donnenfeld et al., 1990. *Am. J. Med. Genet.* 35:529–531. Copyright © 1990 John Wiley & Sons, Inc. Reprinted by permission of Wiley-Liss, Inc.)

CHROMOSOME 8q PARTIAL MONOSOMY

Partial monosomy for 8q is known to result in characteristic findings. Langer-Giedion and tricho-rhino-phalangeal syndromes have been mapped to 8q24. Patients with deletions excluding 8q24 present with clinical manifestations distinct from those seen in Langer-Giedion and tricho-rhino-phalangeal syndromes.

MAIN FEATURES: Growth and psychomotor retardation, carp-shaped mouth, small nose, hypertelorism

ABNORMALITIES

Growth: Growth retardation, short stature

Performance: Psychomotor retardation, developmental delay, poor feeding, abnormal muscle tone

Craniofacies: Round face with prominent forehead, hypertelorism, eye abnormalities, small nose, carp-shaped mouth, micrognathia, abnormal ears, anteverted nares, long philtrum

Limbs: Abnormal hands and feet with abnormal fingers and toes and a single palmar crease

Other: Cardiac defects, respiratory problems

OCCASIONAL ABNORMALITIES: Microcephaly, short neck, hyperextensible joints, hypoplastic thumbs, wide nasal bridge, upward-slanting palpebral fissures, medially thick eyebrows

CLINICAL COURSE: Death in infancy is uncommon.

CYTOGENETICS: Most cases are the result of a de novo defect.

REFERENCES

Donahue ML, Ryan RM. 1995. Interstitial deletion of 8q21 → 22 associated with minor anomalies, congenital heart defect, and Dandy-Walker variant. *Am. J. Med. Genet.* 56:97–100.

Fennell SJ, Benson JW, Kindley AD, Schwarz MJ, Czepulkowski B. 1989. Partial deletion 8q without Langer-Giedion syndrome: a recognisable syndrome. *J. Med. Genet.* 26:167–171.

Fryburg JS, Golden WL. 1993. Interstitial deletion of 8q13.3 → 22.1 associated with craniosynostosis. *Am. J. Med. Genet.* 45:638–641.

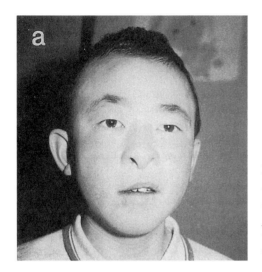

Note sparse hair, prominent ears, medially thick eyebrows, and a pear-shaped nose with prominent columella. (From Yamamoto et al., 1989. *Am. J. Med. Genet.* 32:133–135. Copyright © 1989 John Wiley & Sons, Inc. Reprinted by permission of Wiley-Liss, Inc.)

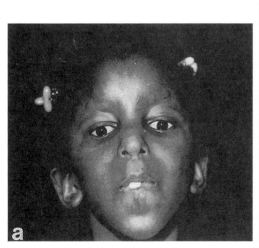
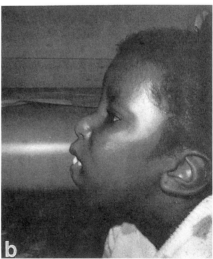

Patient at 6 years. Note pear-shaped nose, thick lips, and prominent ears. Only one of the central upper incisors has erupted. (From Ramos et al., 1992. *Am. J. Med. Genet.* 44:790–794. Copyright © 1992 John Wiley & Sons, Inc. Reprinted by permission of Wiley-Liss, Inc.)

Ramos FJ, McDonald-McGinn DM, Emanuel BS, Zackai EH. 1992. Tricho-rhino-phalangeal syndrome type II (Langer-Giedion) with persistent cloaca and prune belly sequence in a girl with 8q interstitial deletion. *Am. J. Med. Genet.* 44:790–794.

Yamamoto Y, Oguro N, Miyao M, Yanagisawa M. 1989. Tricho-rhino-phalangeal syndrome type I with severe mental retardation due to interstitial deletion of 8q23.3–24.13. *Am. J. Med. Genet.* 32:133–135.

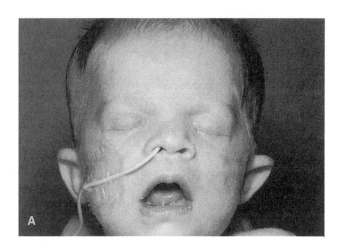

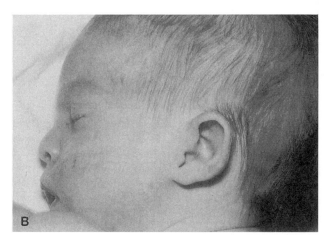

Patient at 2 weeks. Note the carp-shaped mouth, small chin, prominent, apparently low-set ears, hypertelorism, and broad nasal bridge (A). Note the long forehead and facial hypoplasia (B). (From Donahue and Ryan, 1995. *Am. J. Med. Genet.* 56:97–100. Copyright © 1995 John Wiley & Sons, Inc. Reprinted by permission of Wiley-Liss, Inc.)

RING CHROMOSOME 8

Ring chromosome 8 is extremely rare with only a few reported cases. Each patient presented with different clinical manifestations, which are thought to be the result of varying breakpoints and deletions during ring formation. To date, it is impossible to characterize an associated syndrome due to the limited number of patients.

FEATURES

Mental retardation to varying degrees was seen in most patients, as was prenatal onset of growth retardation. Some minor dysmorphic features were also noted, including abnormal skull shape, malformed ears, and thin lips.

REFERENCES

Mingarelli R, Valorani G, Zelante L, Dallapiccola B. 1991. Ring chromosome 8 associated with microcephaly. *Ann. Genet.* 34:90–92.

CHROMOSOME 9p PARTIAL TRISOMY

Partial or complete duplication of chromosome 9p results in a phenotype that is well described. The severity of clinical manifestations is associated with the amount of 9p that is duplicated. Commonly exhibited features include mental retardation, short stature, and characteristic facial features.

MAIN FEATURES: Mental retardation, short stature, bulbous nose, downward-slanting palpebral fissures

ABNORMALITIES

Performance: Developmental delay, mental retardation, hypotonia

Craniofacies: Brachycephaly, large fontaneles, deep-set eyes, hypertelorism, prominent bulbous nose, abnormal nasal bridge, downturned corners of the mouth, abnormal, low-set ears, short/webbed neck, downward-slanting palpebral fissures, abnormal philtrum

Limbs: Single palmar transverse crease, clinodactyly, abnormal fingers and toes with abnormal nails

Other: Widely spaced nipples, joint abnormalities

OCCASIONAL ABNORMALITIES: Syndactyly, highly arched or cleft palate

CLINICAL COURSE: Survival into adulthood has been reported.

CYTOGENETICS: Most cases are the result of familial chromosomal rearrangements, although de novo defects have been documented.

REFERENCES

Bussani Mastellone C, Giovannucci Uzielli ML, Guarducci S, Nathan G. 1991. Four cases of trisomy 9p syndrome with particular chromosome rearrangements. *Ann. Genet.* 34:115–119.

Greig F, Rosenfeld W, Verma RS, Babu KA, David K. 1985. Duplication 11(q22 → qter) in an infant. A case report with review. *Ann. Genet.* 28:185–188.

Haddad BR, Lin AE, Wyandt H, Milunsky A. 1996. Molecular cytogenetic characterisation of the first familial case of partial 9p duplication (p22p24). *J. Med. Genet.* 33:1045–1047.

Motegi T, Watanabe K, Nakamura N, Hasegawa T, Yanagawa Y. 1985. De novo tandem duplication 9p(p12 → p24) with normal GALT activity in red cells. *J. Med. Genet.* 22:64–66.

Petty EM, Gibson LH, Breg WR, Burns JP, Yang-Feng TL. 1993. Mosaic dup (9p) diagnosed by fluorescence in situ hybridization (FISH). *Am. J. Med. Genet.* 45:770–773.

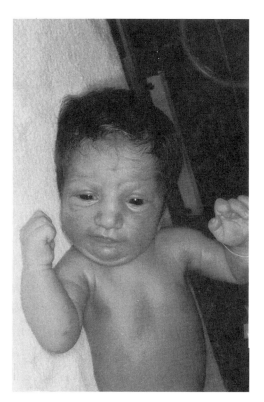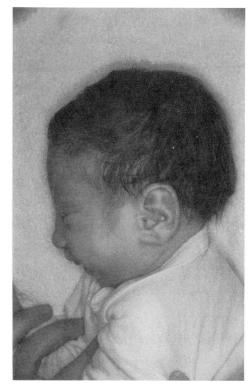

Note brachycephaly, hypertelorism, downward-slanting palpebral fissures, broad, prominent nose, large, low-set ears, and a short neck. (From Bussani Malstellone et al., 1991. *Ann. Genet.* 34:115–119. Reprinted with permission from Expansion Scientifique Francaise.)

CHROMOSOME 9p PARTIAL MONOSOMY

Partial monosomy 9p is a well-described syndrome. A majority of the patients present with mental retardation, trigonocephaly, and other facial dysmorphism. Approximately two-thirds of the cases are de novo with band p22 being the most common site of the breakpoint.

MAIN FEATURES: Mental retardation, trigonocephaly, upward-slanting palpebral fissures, epicanthal folds.

ABNORMALITIES

Performance: Developmental delay, mental retardation, hypotonia

Craniofacies: Trigonocephaly, upward-slanting palpebral fissures, epicanthal folds, hypertelorism, low-set, malformed ears, flat, depressed nasal bridge, anteverted nostrils, long philtrum

Other: Highly arched palate, bilateral clubfoot at birth, short, broad neck, low posterior hairline, widely spaced nipples, umbilical hernia

OCCASIONAL ABNORMALITIES: Strabismus, square hyperconvex fingernails, long fingers and/or toes, thoracic kyphosis, hearing loss

CLINICAL COURSE: Death in infancy is not common.

CYTOGENETICS: Most cases are the result of a de novo defect, although familial chromosomal rearrangements have been documented.

REFERENCES

Cotter PD, Stewart NL. 1990. Partial trisomy 17q and monosomy 9p due to a familial translocation. *Ann. Genet.* 33:231–233.

Giltay JC, Gerssen-Schoorl KB, van der Wagen A. 1994. A case of de novo interstitial deletion of chromosome 9(p12p13). *Clin. Genet.* 46:271–272.

Hoo JJ. 1986. Karyotype-phenotype analysis: 9p deletion versus 10q2 duplication. *Ann. Genet.* 29:266–268.

Shashi V, Golden WL, Fryburg JS. 1994. Choanal atresia in a patient with the deletion (9p) syndrome. *Am. J. Med. Genet.* 49:88–90.

Tayel SM, Kurczynski TW, Casperson S, McCorquodale MM. 1988. Deletion 9p, duplication 18q in two sisters resulting from a maternal (9;18)(p22;q21.3) translocation. *Am. J. Med. Genet.* 31:853–861.

Teebi AS, Gibson L, McGrath J, Meyn MS, Breg WR, Yang-Feng TL. 1993. Molecular and cytogenetic characterization of 9p-abnormalities. *Am. J. Med. Genet.* 46:288–292.

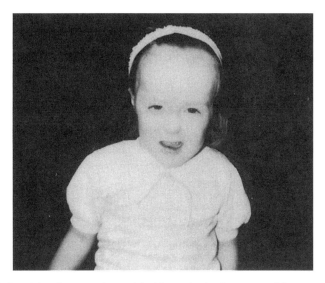

Note the right-sided ptosis, depressed nasal bridge, pinched nose, and long, smooth philtrum. (From Shashi et al., 1994. *Am. J. Med. Genet.* 49:88–90. Copyright © 1994 John Wiley & Sons, Inc. Reprinted by permission of Wiley-Liss, Inc.)

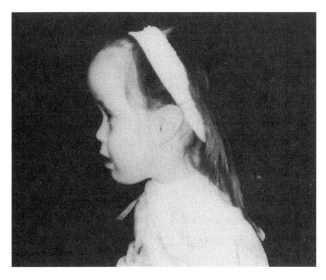

Note striking frontal bossing. (From Shashi et al., 1994. *Am. J. Med. Genet.* 49:88–90. Copyright © 1994 John Wiley & Sons, Inc. Reprinted by permission of Wiley-Liss, Inc.)

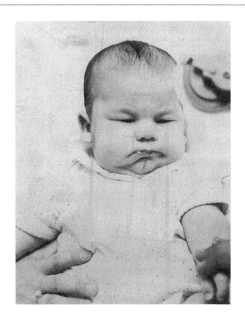

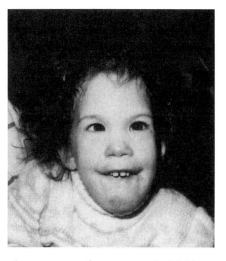

Note long, narrow face, epicanthal folds, telecanthus, and depressed nasal bridge. (From Teebi et al., 1993. *Am. J. Med. Genet.* 46:288–292. Copyright © 1993 John Wiley & Sons, Inc. Reprinted by permission of Wiley-Liss, Inc.)

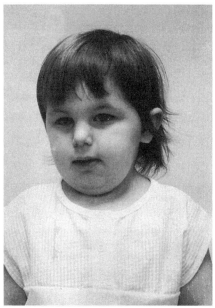

Note prominent lobules of the pinnae, flat, broad nasal bridge, epicanthal folds, and short neck. (From Tayel et al., 1988. *Am. J. Med. Genet.* 31:853–861. Copyright © 1988 John Wiley & Sons, Inc. Reprinted by permission of Wiley-Liss, Inc.)

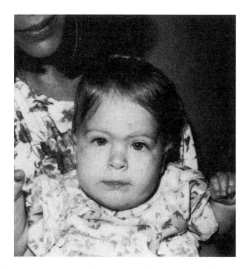

Note narrow forehead, small nose, midface hypoplasia, upward-slanting palpebral fissures, epicanthal folds, thin, long eyebrows, and short neck. (From Teebi et al., 1993. *Am. J. Med. Genet.* 46:288–292. Copyright © 1993 John Wiley & Sons, Inc. Reprinted by permission of Wiley-Liss, Inc.)

CHROMOSOME 9q PARTIAL TRISOMY

Individuals with partial duplications of the long arm of chromosome 9 are very rare. Most of the duplications reported involve the distal portion of 9q. Researchers have concluded that 9q is likely to be involved in the development of the head, neck, and cardiac regions. It has been suggested that this region may also be involved in the manifestation of DiGeorge sequence.

MAIN FEATURES: Mental retardation, failure to thrive, beaked nose

ABNORMALITIES

Growth: Low birth weight, failure to thrive

Performance: Developmental delay, psychomotor retardation, mental retardation, hypotonia

Craniofacies: Microcephaly, dolichocephaly, deep-set eyes, strabismus, beaked nose, prominent nasal bridge, upper lip over lower, retromicrognathia, malformed ears

Genitourinary: Hypoplastic external genitalia

Limbs: Long fingers, slender limbs

Other: Cardiac defects, joint contractures

OCCASIONAL ABNORMALITIES: Bulging forehead, epicanthal folds, small mouth, abnormal fingers and/or toes

CLINICAL COURSE: Death in infancy is uncommon.

CYTOGENETICS: Both de novo defects and familial chromosomal rearrangements have been noted.

REFERENCES

el-Fouly MH, Higgins JV, Kapur S, Sankey BJ, Matisoff DN, Costa-Fox M. 1991. DiGeorge anomaly in an infant with deletion of chromosome 22 and dup(9p) due to adjacent type II disjunction. *Am. J. Med. Genet.* 38:569–573.

Lindgren V, Rosinsky B, Chin J, Berry-Kravis E. 1994. Two patients with overlapping de novo duplications of the long arm of chromosome 9, including one case with Di George sequence. *Am. J. Med. Genet.* 49:67–73.

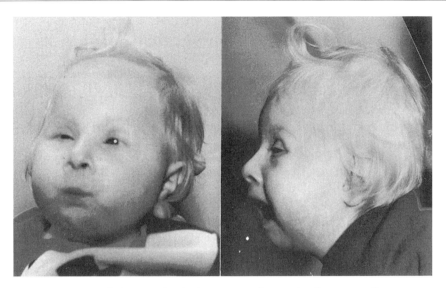

Note deep-set eyes, microphthalmia, beaked nose, small mouth, thin upper lip, retromicrognathia, and pointed chin. (From Lindgren et al., 1994. *Am. J. Med. Genet.* 49:67–73. Copyright © 1994 John Wiley & Sons, Inc. Reprinted by permission of Wiley-Liss, Inc.)

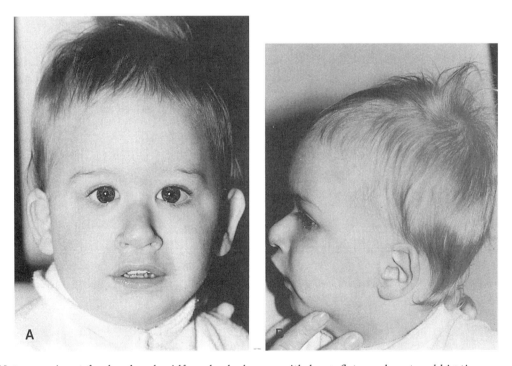

Note prominent forehead and midface, beaked nose, with long, flat nasal root and big tip, bilateral epicanthic folds, convergent strabismus, micrognathia, and underfolded ears. (From Stalker et al., 1993. *Am. J. Med. Genet.* 45:456–459. Copyright © 1993 John Wiley & Sons, Inc. Reprinted by permission of Wiley-Liss, Inc.)

Spinner NB, Lucas JN, Poggensee M, Jacquette M, Schneider A. 1993. Duplication 9q34 → qter identified by chromosome painting. *Am. J. Med. Genet.* 45:609–613.

Stalker HJ, Ayme S, Delneste D, Scarpelli H, Vekemans M, Der Kaloustian VM. 1993. Duplication of 9q12–q33: a case report and implications for the dup(9q) syndrome. *Am. J. Med. Genet.* 45:456–459.

Yamamoto Y, Oguro N, Nara T, Horita H, Niitsu N, Imaizumi S. 1988. Duplication of part of 9q due to maternal 12;9 inverted insertion associated with pyloric stenosis. *Am. J. Med. Genet.* 31:379–384.

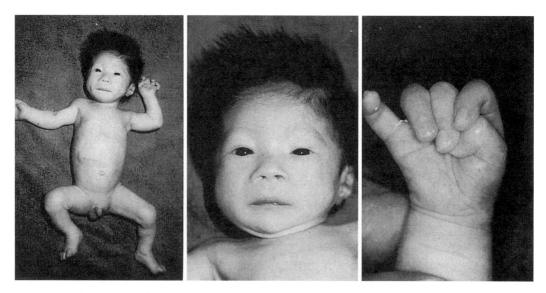

Note round face, broad, flared nose, long philtrum, thin upper lip, mild micrognathia, low-set ears, and adducted thumb. (From Yamamoto et al., 1988. *Am. J. Med. Genet.* 31:379–384. Copyright © 1988 John Wiley & Sons, Inc. Reprinted by permission of Wiley-Liss, Inc.)

CHROMOSOME 9q PARTIAL MONOSOMY

Chromosome 9q partial deletion is rare with no clearly defined syndrome.

MAIN FEATURES: Hypotonia, eye anomalies, abnormal skull shape, downward-slanting palpebral fissures

ABNORMALITIES

Growth: Growth retardation

Performance: Developmental delay, psychomotor retardation, hypotonia

Eyes: Strabismus, ptosis, nystagmus, fovial hypoplasia, colobomas

Craniofacies: Abnormal head shape (i.e., brachycephaly), downward-slanting palpebral fissures, small, thin nose, low-set, malformed ears, increased inner canthal distance, epicanthal folds, abnormal mouth size, high-arched palate, cleft palate, flat nasal bridge

Other: Dilated ventricles, digital malformations, congenital heart defects

OCCASIONAL ABNORMALITIES: Seizures, umbilical hernia

CLINICAL COURSE: Life into teens reported

CYTOGENETICS: Most patients represent de novo defects.

REFERENCES

Farrell SA, Siegel-Bartelt J, Teshima I. 1991. Patients with deletions of 9q22q34 do not define a syndrome: three case reports and a literature review. *Clin. Genet.* 40:207–214.

Kroes HY, Tuerlings JH, Hordijk R, Folkers NR, ten Kate LP. 1994. Another patient with an interstitial deletion of chromosome 9: case report and a review of six cases with del(9)(q22q32). *J. Med. Genet.* 31:156–158.

Pfeiffer RA, Lachmann E, Schreyer W, Volleth M. 1993. Deletion of 9q22: a new observation suggesting a specific phenotype. *Ann. Genet.* 36:167–170.

Schimmenti LA, Berry SA, Tuchman M, Hirsch B. 1994. Infant with multiple congenital anomalies and deletion (9)(q34.3). *Am. J. Med. Genet.* 51:140–142.

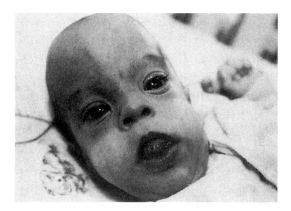

Patient at age 5 months. Note dolichocephaly, bilateral epicanthal folds, eyelid hemangiomata, and upturned nose. (From Schimmenti et al., 1994. *Am. J. Med. Genet.* 51:140–142. Copyright © 1994 John Wiley & Sons, Inc. Reprinted by permission of Wiley-Liss, Inc.)

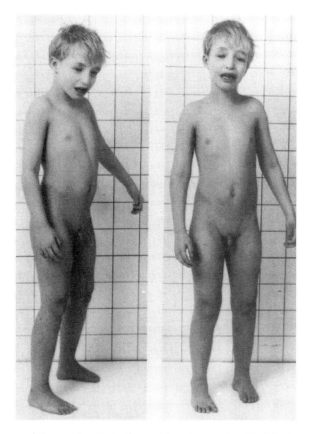

Patient at age 9 years and 6 months. Note frontal bossing, epicanthal folds, small ears, hypoplastic scrotum, and small penis. (From Kroes et al., 1994. *J. Med. Genet.* 31:156–158. Reprinted with permission from BMJ Publishing Group.)

RING CHROMOSOME 9

Individuals presenting with ring chromosome 9 are extremely rare. Due to the limited number of reported cases, a definitive syndrome has yet to be defined. Some researchers have reported that patients with ring chromosme 9 manifest features similar to those exhibited in partial del(9p).

MAIN FEATURES: Mental retardation, trigonocephaly, anteverted nostrils, upward-slanting palpebral fissures

ABNORMALITIES

Growth: Growth retardation

Performance: Mental retardation, psychomotor retardation

Craniofacies: Microcephaly, trigonocephaly, arched or prominent eyebrows, upward-slanting palpebral fissures, exophthalmia, anteverted nostrils, long philtrum, abnormal mouth, micrognathia, malformed, low-set ears, abnormal nose

Genitourinary: Abnormal testes

Other: Strabismus, high-arched palate, cardiac defects, widely spaced nipples

OCCASIONAL ABNORMALITIES: Hypertelorism, short neck, long, slender fingers, seizures

CLINICAL COURSE: Death in infancy is uncommon. Survival into adulthood is documented.

CYTOGENETICS: Usually the result of a de novo defect

REFERENCES

Dipierri JE, Matayoshi T. 1982. Ring chromosome 9: identification of a new case by G- and C-banding. *Ann. Genet.* 25:243–245.

Fraisse J, Lauras B, Ooghe MJ, Freycon F, Rethore MO. 1974. [A case of annular chromosome 9. Identification by controlled denaturation]. *Ann. Genet.* 17:175–180.

Leung AK, Rudd NL. 1988. A case of ring (9)/del(9p) mosaicism associated with gastroesophageal reflux. *Am. J. Med. Genet.* 29:43–48.

Nakajima S, Yanagisawa M, Kamoshita S, Nakagome Y. 1976. Mental retardation and congenital malformations associated with a ring chromosome 9. *Hum. Genet.* 32:289–293.

Smith A, Evans WA, Woolnough H. 1989. Post mortem studies on two patients with 1–2 band cytogenetic deletions: 10q26 → qter and r(9)(p24q34). *Ann. Genet.* 32:220–224.

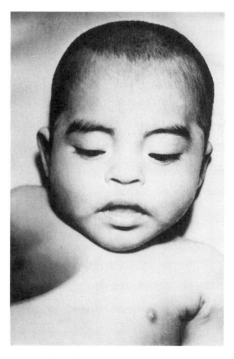 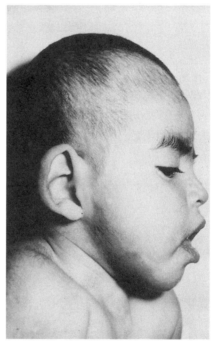

Note the arched and prominent eyebrows, upward-slanting palpebral fissures, epicanthal folds, short nose, long, flat nasal bridge, and long philtrum. (From Dipierri et al., 1982. *Ann. Genet.* 25:243–245. Reprinted with permission from Expansion Scientifique Francaise.)

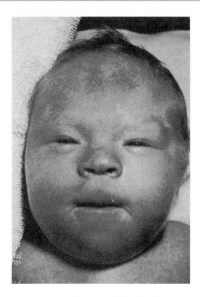

Note upward-slanting palpebral fissures, epicanthal folds, flat nasal bridge, anteverted nares, long philtrum, thin lips, and nevus flammeus on the forehead. (From Leung and Rudd, 1988. *Am. J. Med. Genet.* 29:43–48. Copyright © 1988 John Wiley & Sons, Inc. Reprinted by permission of Wiley-Liss, Inc.)

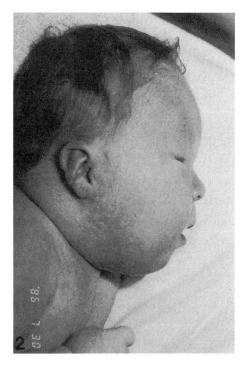

Note brachycephaly, apparently short neck with redundant posterior skin, apparently low-set, hypoplastic auricles, and micrognathia. (From Leung and Rudd, 1988. *Am. J. Med. Genet.* 29:43–48. Copyright © 1988 John Wiley & Sons, Inc. Reprinted by permission of Wiley-Liss, Inc.)

CHROMOSOME 10p PARTIAL TRISOMY

Partial trisomy 10p results in a predictable pattern of malformations. Patients with this defect almost always present with craniofacial abnormalities, growth and mental retardation, and various skeletal abnormalities. The vast majority of these patients result from familial chromosomal rearrangements.

MAIN FEATURES: Low-set, malformed ears, frontal bossing, growth and mental retardation

ABNORMALITIES

Growth: Growth retardation

Performance: Psychomotor retardation, developmental delay, mental retardation, failure to thrive, hypotonia

Craniofacies: Frontal bossing, dolichocephaly, low-set, malformed ears, abnormal nasal bridge, sagging cheeks

Genitourinary: Hypoplastic genitalia

Other: Heart murmur, abnormal hands and feet

OCCASIONAL ABNORMALITIES: Turtle beak mouth, cleft lip and/or palate, renal malformations, abducted, flexed lower limbs, clubfoot.

CLINICAL COURSE: Death in infancy is uncommon.

CYTOGENETICS: Most cases are the result of familial chromosomal rearrangements.

REFERENCES

Kozma C, Meck JM. 1994. Familial 10p trisomy resulting from a maternal pericentric inversion. *Am. J. Med. Genet.* 49:281–287.

Ohba K, Ohdo S, Sonoda T. 1990. Trisomy 10p syndrome owing to maternal pericentric inversion. *J. Med. Genet.* 27:264–266.

Stone D, Ning Y, Guan XY, Kaiser-Kupfer M, Wynshaw-Boris A, Biesecker L. 1996. Characterization of familial partial 10p trisomy by chromosomal microdissection, FISH, and microsatellite dosage analysis. *Hum. Genet.* 98:396–402.

Wiktor A, Feldman GL, Kratkoczki P, Ditmars DM Jr, Van Dyke DL. 1994. 10p duplication characterized by fluorescence in situ hybridization. *Am. J. Med. Genet.* 52:315–318.

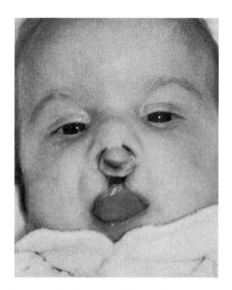

Patient at 4 months. Note wide nasal bridge and bilateral cleft lip and palate. (From Wiktor et al., 1994. *Am. J. Med. Genet.* 52:315–318. Copyright © 1994 John Wiley & Sons, Inc. Reprinted by permission of Wiley-Liss, Inc.)

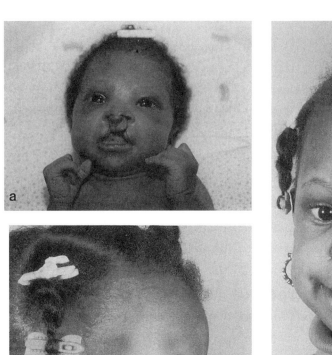
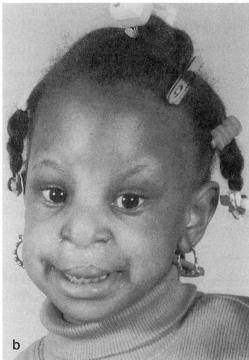
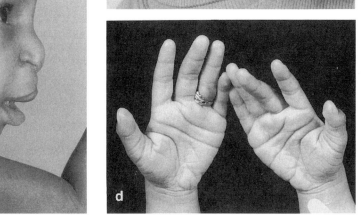

Patient at 2 weeks (a). Note sloping forehead and hyperflexed position of upper limbs. Patient at 4 years (b,c). Note broad nasal bridge, upward-slanted palpebral fissures, round saggy cheeks, protruding maxilla, and turtle beak mouth. Photograph of patient's palms (d). Note the extra transverse creases and the increased length of the palm. (From Kozma and Meck, 1994. *Am. J. Med. Genet.* 49:281–287. Copyright © 1994 John Wiley & Sons, Inc. Reprinted by permission of Wiley-Liss, Inc.)

CHROMOSOME 10p PARTIAL MONOSOMY

Although uncommon, patients with partial deletion of 10p are known to present with characteristic findings. Deletion of 10p13 has been linked to hypoparathyroidism and DiGeorge sequence. Many of the phenotypic manifestations of partial 10p deletion are similar to those seen in Velocardio facial/DiGeorge syndromes.

MAIN FEATURES: Mental retardation, abnormally shaped skull, hypertelorism, dysplastic, small, low-set ears

ABNORMALITIES

Growth: Growth retardation

Performance: Psychomotor retardation, mental retardation

Craniofacies: Abnormally shaped skull, downward-slanting palpebral fissures, epicanthal folds, hypertelorism, low nasal bridge, micrognathia, and dysplastic, small, low-set ears

Other: Cardiac defects, short neck, abnormal hands and feet

OCCASIONAL ABNORMALITIES: Anteverted nostrils, frontal bossing, genital abnormalities, urinary tract anomalies, hearing loss, abnormal fingers and toes, simian creases, clinodactyly, widely spaced nipples

CLINICAL COURSE: Death in infancy is not common.

CYTOGENETICS: Most cases are the result of a de novo defect, although familial chromosomal rearrangements have been documented.

REFERENCES

Dasouki M, Jurecic V, Phillips JA 3rd, Whitlock JA, Baldini A. 1997. DiGeorge anomaly and chromosome 10p deletions: one or two loci? *Am. J. Med. Genet.* 73:72–75.

Lipson A, Fagan K, Colley A, Colley P, Sholler G, Issacs D, Oates RK. 1996. Velo-cardio-facial and partial DiGeorge phenotype in a child with interstitial deletion at 10p13—implications for cytogenetics and molecular biology. *Am. J. Med. Genet.* 65:304–308.

Obregon MG, Mingarelli R, Giannotti A, di Comite A, Spedicato FS, Dallapiccola B. 1992. Partial deletion 10p syndrome: report of two patients. *Ann. Genet.* 35:101–104.

Schuffenhauer S, Seidel H, Oechsler H, Belohradsky B, Bernsau U, Murken J, Meitinger T. 1995. DiGeorge syndrome and partial monosomy 10p: case report and review. *Ann. Genet.* 38, no. 3:162–167.

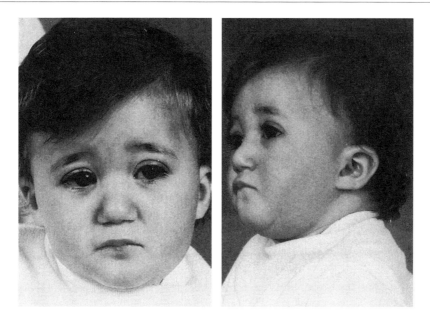

Patient at 1 year and 6 months. Note deficient alae nasi, almond-shaped palpebral fissures, bulbous nasal tip, and small dysplastic ears. (From Lipson et al., 1996. *Am. J. Med. Genet.* 65:304–308. Copyright © 1996 John Wiley & Sons, Inc. Reprinted by permission of Wiley-Liss, Inc.)

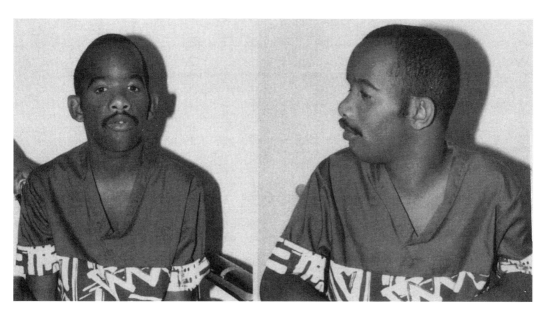

Patient at 15 years and 6 months. Note hypertelorism, epicanthal folds, and frontal bossing. (From Dasouki et al., 1997. *Am. J. Med. Genet.* 73:72–75. Copyright © 1997 John Wiley & Sons, Inc. Reprinted by permission of Wiley-Liss, Inc.)

Shapira M, Borochowitz Z, Bar-El H, Dar H, Etzioni A, Lorber A. 1994. Deletion of the short arm of chromosome 10(10p13): report of a patient and review. *Am. J. Med. Genet.* 52:34–38.

Tokano T, Horigome H, Shibata S. 1993. Exclusion map of the gene for neuraminidase from 10(pter → p15.1). *Clin. Genet.* 43:166–167.

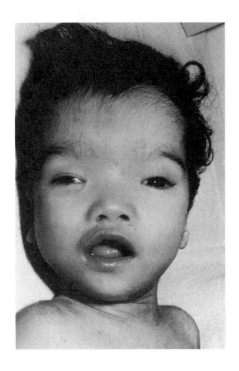

Patient at 2 years. Note microcephaly, hypertelorism, epicanthal folds, strabismus, and micrognathia. (From Takano et al., 1993. *Clin. Genet.* 43:166–167. Copyright © 1993 Munksgaard International Publishers Ltd., Copenhagen, Denmark, with permission.)

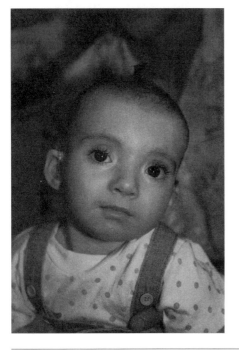

Patient at 1 year and 8 months. Note hypertelorism, low nasal bridge, micrognathia, and dysmorphic, low-set ears. (From Schuffenhauer et al., 1995. *Ann. Genet.* 38:162–167. Reprinted with permission from Expansion Scientifique Francaise.)

CHROMOSOME 10q PARTIAL TRISOMY

Some researchers have suggested that partial trisomy 10q results in a recognizable pattern of malformations. Other researchers have concluded that it is not yet possible to delineate a syndrome. The variation exhibited is likely the result of different 10q breakpoints among patients or due to a partial duplication, partial deletion syndrome. A majority of partial 10q+ patients are trisomic for the distal one-third of 10q, but differences in band involvement are documented.

MAIN FEATURES: Microcephaly, deep-set, small eyes, developmental delay, growth retardation

ABNORMALITIES

Growth: Growth retardation

Performance: Developmental delay, mental retardation, hypotonia

Craniofacies: Microcephaly, high, prominent forehead, deep-set, small eyes, upturned nose, bow-shaped mouth, micrognathia, prominent philtrum, low-set ears

Other: Abnormal fingers and toes

OCCASIONAL ABNORMALITIES: Respiratory distress, epicanthal folds, flat, thick ear helix, slender limbs, hypertelorism

CLINICAL COURSE: Death in infancy is uncommon.

CYTOGENETICS: Most cases are the result of familial chromosomal rearrangements.

REFERENCES

Aalfs CM, Hoovers JM, Nieste-Otter MA, Mannens MM, Hennekam RC, Leschot NJ. 1995. Further delineation of the partial proximal trisomy 10q syndrome. *J. Med. Genet.* 32:968–971.

Boon C, Markello T, Jackson-Cook C, Pandya A. 1996. Partial trisomy 10 mosaicism with cutaneous manifestations: report of a case and review of the literature. *Clin. Genet.* 50:417–421.

Briscioli V, Floridia G, Rossi E, Selicorni A, Lalatta F, Zuffardi O. 1993. Trisomy 10qter confirmed by in situ hybridisation. *J. Med. Genet.* 30:601–603.

de Michelena MI, Campos PJ. 1991. A new case of proximal 10q partial trisomy. *J. Med. Genet.* 28:205–206.

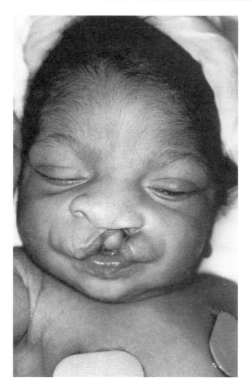

Patient at birth. Note thick, curly hair, high, prominent forehead, prominent nasal root, hypertelorism, cleft lip, and micrognathia. (From Boon et al., 1996. *Clin. Genet.* 50:417–421. Copyright © 1996 Munksgaard International Publishers Ltd., Copenhagen, Denmark, with permission.)

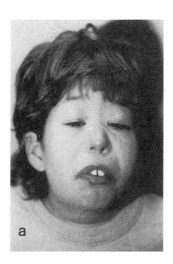
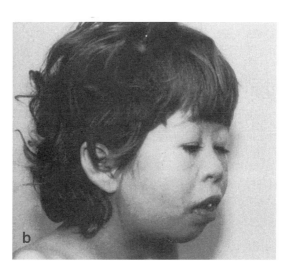

Note flat facial profile, ptosis, and blepharophimosis. (From Johnson and Sutliff, 1994. *Am. J. Med. Genet.* 52:184–187. Copyright © 1994 John Wiley & Sons, Inc. Reprinted by permission of Wiley-Liss, Inc.)

Hoo JJ, Chao M, Szego K, Rauer M, Echiverri SC, Harris C. 1995. Four new cases of inverted terminal duplication: a modified hypothesis of mechanism of origin. *Am. J. Med. Genet.* 58:299–304.

Johnson VP, Sutliff WC. 1994. Duplication 10q confirmed by DNA in situ hybridization. *Am. J. Med. Genet.* 52:184–187.

Pfeiffer RA, Junemann A, Lorenz B, Sieber E. 1995. Aplasia of the optic nerve in two cases of partial trisomy 10q24-ter. *Clin. Genet.* 48:183–187.

Tonk V, Schneider NR, Delgado MR, Mao J, Schultz RA. 1996. Identification and molecular confirmation of a small chromosome 10q duplication [dir dup(10)(q24.2 → q24.3)] inherited from a mother mosaic for the abnormality. *Am. J. Med. Genet.* 61:16–20.

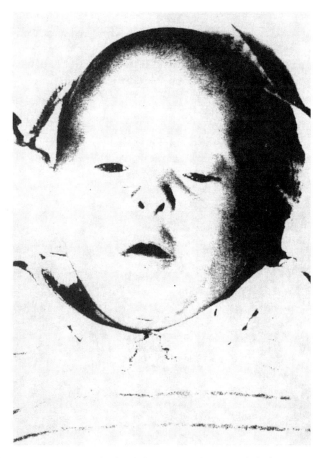

Patient at 2 months. Note narrow palpebral fissures and microphthalmia. (From Pfeiffer et al., 1995. *Clin. Genet.* 48:183–187. Copyright © 1995 Munksgaard International Publishers Ltd., Copenhagen, Denmark, with permission.)

CHROMOSOME 10q PARTIAL MONOSOMY

Partial deletions of the q arm of chromosome 10 are not common.

MAIN FEATURES: Psychomotor retardation, hypotonia, telecanthus/hypertelorism, low-set, malformed ears, broad nasal bridge

ABNORMALITIES

Growth: Growth retardation

Performance: Hypotonia, psychomotor retardation, developmental delay

Eyes: Strabismus, telecanthus/hypertelorism

Craniofacies: Low-set, malformed ears, broad nasal bridge, broad, prominent forehead, small or large nose, long, prominent filtrum, thin lips

Other: Heart murmur, ventricular septal defect (VSD), urogenital defects

OCCASIONAL ABNORMALITIES: Hypertonia, short neck, plagiocephaly, dolichocephaly, microcephaly, upward-slanting palpebral fissures, small chin, digit abnormalities, nipple anomalies

CLINICAL COURSE: Life into adulthood has been reported.

CYTOGENETICS: Most cases are the result of a de novo defect, but some result from a familial chromosomal rearrangement

REFERENCES

Borovik CL, Brunoni D. 1991. Terminal deletion of chromosome 10q26 due to a paternal translocation [(7;10)(q36;q26)]. *Am. J. Med. Genet.* 41:534–536.

Chung YP, Hwa HL, Tseng LH, Shyu MK, Lee CN, Shih JC, Hsieh FJ. 1998. Prenatal diagnosis of monosomy 10q25 associated with single umbilical artery and sex reversal: report of a case. *Prenat. Diagn.* 18:73–77.

Costakos DT, Love LA, Josephson K, Sekhon G. 1998. Pathological case of the month. Chromosome 10 qter deletion syndrome. *Arch. Pediatr. Adolesc. Med.* 152:507–508.

Farrell SA, Szymonowicz W, Chow G, Summers AM. 1993. Interstitial deletion of chromosome 10q23: a new case and review. *J. Med. Genet.* 30:248–250.

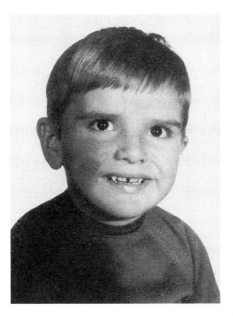

Patient at age 7 years. Note deep-set eyes, telecanthus, wide mouth with downturned corners. (From Fryns et al., 1991. *Am. J. Med. Genet.* 40:343–344. Copyright © 1991 John Wiley & Sons, Inc. Reprinted by permission of Wiley-Liss, Inc.)

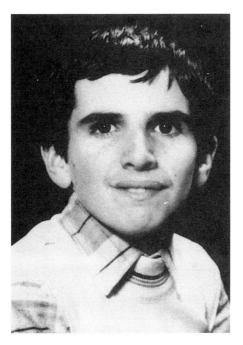

Patient at age 22 years. Note deeply sunken eyes and slender nose. (From Fryns et al., 1991. *Am. J. Med. Genet.* 40:343–344. Copyright © 1991 John Wiley & Sons, Inc. Reprinted by permission of Wiley-Liss, Inc.)

Fewtrell MS, Tam PK, Thomson AH, Fitchett M, Currie J, Huson SM, Mulligan LM. 1994. Hirschsprung's disease associated with a deletion of chromosome 10(q11.2q21.2): a further link with the neurocristopathies? *J. Med. Genet.* 31:325–327.

Fryns JP, Bulcke J, Verdu P, Carton H, Kleczkowska A, Van den Berghe H. 1991. Apparent late-onset Cockayne syndrome and interstitial deletion of the long arm of chromosome 10(del(10)(q11.23q21.2)). *Am. J. Med. Genet.* 40:343–344.

Lobo S, Cervenka J, London A, Pierpont ME. 1992. Interstitial deletion of 10q: clinical features and literature review. *Am. J. Med. Genet.* 43:701–703.

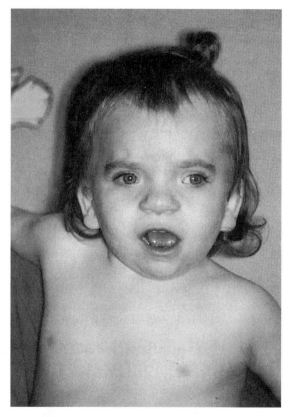

Patient at 2 years. Note broad forehead, broad nasal root, divergent strabismus, prominent philtrum, thin, bow-shaped upper lip, and thick pinnae. (From Lobo et al., 1992. *Am. J. Med. Genet.* 43:701–703. Copyright © 1992 John Wiley & Sons, Inc. Reprinted by permission of Wiley-Liss, Inc.)

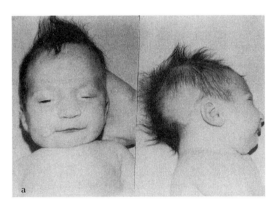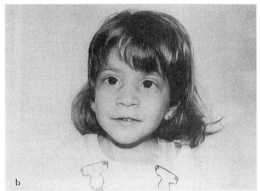

Patient at birth (a) and at age 4 years (b). Note microcephaly, prominent forehead, downward-slanting palpebral fissures, small nose, broad nasal bridge, long philtrum, thin upper lip, and small chin. (From Borovik and Brunoni, 1991. *Am. J. Med. Genet.* 41:534–536. Copyright © 1991 John Wiley & Sons, Inc. Reprinted by permission of Wiley-Liss, Inc.)

RING CHROMOSOME 10

Ring chromosome 10 is a very rare cytogenetic finding. As is common in many patients with ring chromosomes, mental and growth retardation are often exhibited. In general, ring chromosomes are extremely unstable, resulting in tissue mosaicism. It has been suggested that this mosaicism may be responsible for tumorigenesis or abnormal fetal development, especially when the function of genes in these pathways is disturbed.

MAIN FEATURES: Microcephaly, hypertelorism, growth retardation, mental retardation

ABNORMALITIES

Growth: Growth retardation

Performance: Mental retardation and poor feeding

Craniofacies: Microcephaly, malformed, low-set ears, hypertelorism, long philtrum, micrognathia

Genitourinary: Abnormal genitalia

Other: Strabismus and gap between the hallux and second toe

CLINICAL COURSE: Death in infancy is uncommon.

CYTOGENETICS: Usually the result of a de novo defect

REFERENCES

Blennow E, Tillberg E. 1996. Small extra ring chromosome derived from chromosome 10p: clinical report and characterisation by FISH. *J. Med. Genet.* 33:399–402.

Calabrese G, Franchi PG, Stuppia L, Mingarelli R, Rossi C, Ramenghi L, Marino M, Morizio E, Peila R, Antonucci A, et al. 1994. A newborn with ring chromosome 10, aganglionic megacolon, and renal hypoplasia. *J. Med. Genet.* 31:804–806.

Kondo I, Shimakura Y, Hirano T, Kaneko M, Yabuta K. 1984. Ring chromosome 10 syndrome: case report and the possibility of clinical diagnosis. *Clin. Genet.* 25:196–200.

Nakai H, Adachi M, Katsushima N, Yamazaki N, Sakamoto M, Tada K. 1983. Ring chromosome 10 and its clinical features. *J. Med. Genet.* 20:142–144.

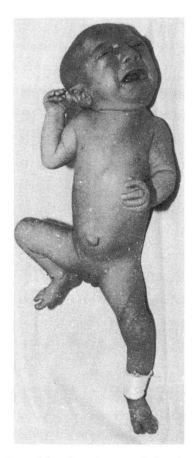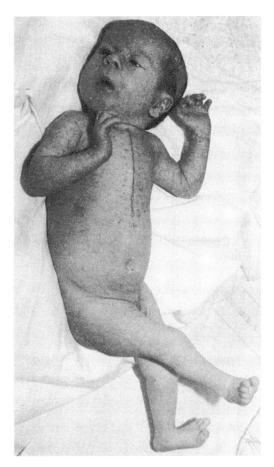

Note frontal bossing, downward-slanting palpebral fissures, mildly stubby nose, large nares, long philtrum, thin lips, and micrognathia. (From Calabrese et al., 1994. *J. Med. Genet.* 31:804–806. Reprinted with permission from BMJ Publishing Group.)

CHROMOSOME 11p PARTIAL TRISOMY

Patients with partial trisomy for 11p present with variable features. Phenotypic manifestations appear to be correlated with the location of the duplication. Research has demonstrated an association of Beckwith–Wiedemann syndrome (BWS) with trisomy 11p15. Additionally, in some cases, BWS appears to result from paternal disomy for 11p15.5. Due to the limited number of patients and the clinical variability, it has not been possible to characterize a syndrome for partial trisomy of 11p.

MAIN FEATURES: Broad, flat nasal bridge, hypertelorism, growth retardation

ABNORMALITIES

Growth: Growth retardation

Craniofacies: Flat, broad nasal bridge, hypertelorism, cleft lip and/or palate, macroglossia

OCCASIONAL ABNORMALITIES: Abnormal muscle tone, nystagmus, seizures, psychomotor retardation

CLINICAL COURSE: Death in infancy is common.

CYTOGENETICS: Both familial chromosomal rearrangements and de novo defects have been reported.

REFERENCES

Aalfs CM, Fantes JA, Wenniger-Prick LJ, Sluijter S, Hennekam RC, van Heyningen V, Hoovers JM. 1997. Tandem duplication of 11p12–p13 in a child with borderline development delay and eye abnormalities: dose effect of the PAX6 gene product? *Am. J. Med. Genet.* 73:267–271.

Drut RM, Drut R. 1996. Nonimmune fetal hydrops and placentomegaly: diagnosis of familial Wiedemann-Beckwith syndrome with trisomy 11p15 using FISH. *Am. J. Med. Genet.* 62:145–149.

Speleman F, Mannens M, Redeker B, Vercruyssen M, Van Oostveldt P, Leroy J, Slater R. 1991. Characterization of a de novo duplication of 11p14 → p13, using fluorescent in situ hybridization and southern hybridization. *Cytogenet. Cell. Genet.* 56:129–131.

Turleau C, de Grouchy J, Chavin-Colin F, Martelli H, Voyer M, Charlas R. 1984. Trisomy 11p15 and Beckwith-Wiedemann syndrome. A report of two cases. *Hum. Genet.* 67:219–221.

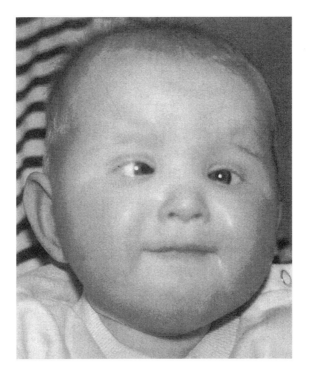

Patient at 5 months. Note the mild midface hypoplasia, small and deep-set eyes, strabismus, broad nasal bridge, and small mouth. (From Aalfs et al., 1997. *Am. J. Med. Genet.* 73:267–271. Copyright © 1997 John Wiley & Sons, Inc. Reprinted by permission of Wiley-Liss, Inc.)

CHROMOSOME 11p PARTIAL MONOSOMY

Individuals with partial monosomy for 11p often present with characteristics that include biparietal foramina and multiple exostoses. Additional research has been successful in mapping the gene for autosomal dominant multiple exostoses to 11p. Other investigators have mapped a Wilms tumor gene to 11p. The WAGR syndrome associated with 11p13 deletion represents a prime example of a contiguous gene syndrome.

MAIN FEATURES: Biparietal foramina, multiple exostoses, mental retardation

ABNORMALITIES

Performance: Mental retardation, developmental delay

Craniofacies: Biparietal foramina, large fontanelles, brachycephaly, short philtrum

Other: Multiple exostoses

OCCASIONAL ABNORMALITIES: Adipose appearance, hypotonia, simian crease, micropenis and other genital abnormalities

CLINICAL COURSE: Death in infancy is not common; survival into adulthood is reported.

CYTOGENETICS: Both de novo defects and familial chromosomal rearrangements have been documented.

REFERENCES

Bartsch O, Wuyts W, Van Hul W, Hecht JT, Meinecke P, Hogue D, Werner W, Zabel B, Hinkel GK, Powell CM, Shaffer LG, Willems PJ. 1996. Delineation of a contiguous gene syndrome with multiple exostoses, enlarged parietal foramina, craniofacial dysostosis, and mental retardation, caused by deletions in the short arm of chromosome 11. *Am. J. Hum. Genet.* 58:734–742.

Hahnemann JM, Vejerslev LO. 1997. Accuracy of cytogenetic findings on chorionic villus sampling (CVS)—diagnostic consequences of CVS mosaicism and non-mosaic discrepancy in centres contributing to EUCROMIC 1986–1992. *Prenat. Diagn.* 17:801–820.

Huff V, Miwa H, Haber DA, Call KM, Housman D, Strong LC, Saunders GF. 1991. Evidence for WT1 as a Wilms tumor (WT) gene: intragenic germinal deletion in bilateral WT. *Am. J. Hum. Genet.* 48:997–1003.

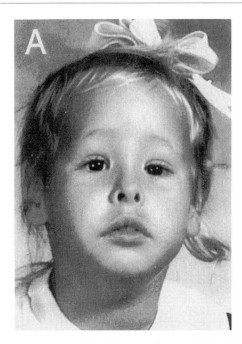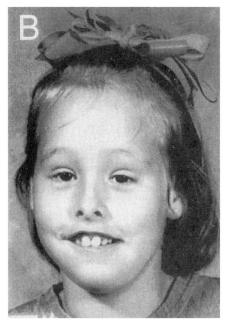

Patient at 4 years (A). Patient at 8 years (B). Note bilateral epicanthal folds, ptosis, short philtrum, and downturned lip. (From Potocki and Shaffer, 1996. *Am. J. Med. Genet.* 62:319–325. Copyright © 1996 John Wiley & Sons, Inc. Reprinted by permission of Wiley-Liss, Inc.)

Ligon AH, Potocki L, Shaffer LG, Stickens D, Evans GA. 1998. Gene for multiple exostoses (EXT2) maps to 11(p11.2p12) and is deleted in patients with a contiguous gene syndrome. *Am. J. Med. Genet.* 75:538–540.

McGaughran JM, Ward HB, Evans DG. 1995. WAGR syndrome and multiple exostoses in a patient with del(11)(p11.2p14.2) *J. Med. Genet.* 32:823–824.

Potocki L, Shaffer LG. 1996. Interstitial deletion of 11(p11.2p12): a newly described contiguous gene deletion syndrome involving the gene for hereditary multiple exostoses (EXT2). *Am. J. Med. Genet.* 62:319–325.

Shaffer LG, Hecht JT, Ledbetter DH, Greenberg F. 1993. Familial interstitial deletion 11(p11.12p12) associated with parietal foramina, brachymicrocephaly, and mental retardation. *Am. J. Med. Genet.* 45:581–583.

CHROMOSOME 11q PARTIAL TRISOMY

In adults, duplication of chromosome 11q can imitate Pitt–Rogers–Danks syndrome.

MAIN FEATURES: Micrognathia, hypertelorism, micropenis, large ears

ABNORMALITIES

Performance: Developmental delay, mental retardation, hypotonia

Eyes: Hypertelorism

Craniofacies: Micrognathia, large, low-set ears, retracted lower lip, short nose, long philtrum

Other: Spina bifida, congenital heart defects, micropenis

CLINICAL COURSE: A 50-year-old woman is reported.

CYTOGENETICS: Most patients result from a familial chromosomal translocation

REFERENCES

de Die-Smulders CE, Engelen JJ. 1996. 11Q duplication in a patient with Pitt–Rogers–Danks phenotype. *Am. J. Med. Genet.* 66:116–117.

Park JP, McDermet MK, Doody AM, Marin-Padilla JM, Moeschler JB, Wurster-Hill DH. 1993. Familial t(11;13)(q21;q14) and the duplication 11q, 13q phenotype. *Am. J. Med. Genet.* 45:46–48.

Pfeiffer RA, Schutz C. 1993. Tandem duplication 11q23-ter in the dysmorphic child of a retarded mother mosaic for the same anomaly with no apparent abnormalities. *Ann. Genet.* 36:163–166.

Takano T, Yamanouchi Y, Kawashima S, Date M, Hashira S, Kida M, Abe T, Nakahori Y, Nakagome Y. 1993. 11q trisomy detected by fluorescence in situ hybridization. *Clin. Genet.* 44:324–328.

Wenger SL, Steele MW, Boone LY, Lenkey SG, Cummins JH, Chen XQ. 1995. "Balanced" karyotypes in six abnormal offspring of balanced reciprocal translocation normal carrier parents. *Am. J. Med. Genet.* 55:47–52.

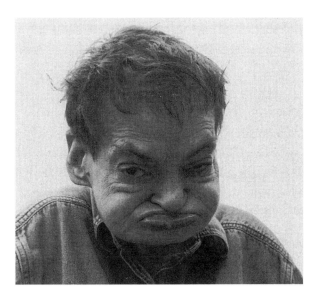

Patient at age 50 years. Note prominent eyes, hypertelorism, tip of the nose overriding the upper lip, and the everted lower lip. (From Die-Smulders, 1996. *Am. J. Med. Genet.* 66:116–117, with permission.)

CHROMOSOME 11q PARTIAL MONOSOMY
Jacobsen Syndrome

Over 50 cases of this syndrome have been reported. The majority involve deletion 11q23 → qter. It is thought that the band responsible for the clinical features is 11q24.1. Seventy-five percent of affected individuals are female.

MAIN FEATURES: Trigonocephaly, congenital heart defects, downturned mouth

ABNORMALITIES

Growth: Prenatal and postnatal growth retardation

Performance: Mental retardation, developmental delay, hypotonia leading to spasticity

Eye: Hypertelorism, ptosis, strabismus, epicanthus

Craniofacies: Trigonocephaly, microcephaly, downturned mouth, abnormal palpebral slant, low-set, malformed ears, short nose, high forehead, epicanthal folds, high-arched palate, depressed nasal bridge, micrognathia

Other: Congenital heart defects, brain abnormalities, bilateral simian creases, urogenital defects, hand and foot abnormalities, pancytopenia/thrombocytopenia, joint contractures

OCCASIONAL ABNORMALITIES: Ventriculomegaly, bulbous nasal tip, retrognathia, abnormal teeth alignment, inguinal hernia, clinodactyly, syndactyly, pyloric stenosis, cleft lip/palate, colobomas, hydrocephalus, renal malformations, macrocephaly

CLINICAL COURSE: Life can be limited if there is a severe cardiac defect. Otherwise life expactancy is normal.

CYTOGENETICS: Most patients result from a familial chromosomal translocation

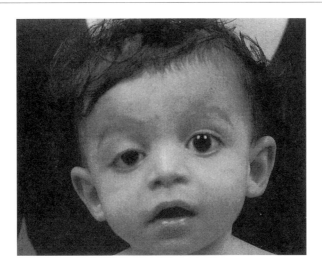

Patient at age 4.5 months. Note brachycephaly, facial asymmetry, ptosis, and downward-slanting palpebral fissures. (From Lewanda et al., 1995. *Am. J. Med. Genet.* 59:193–198. Copyright © 1995 John Wiley & Sons, Inc. Reprinted by permission of Wiley-Liss, Inc.)

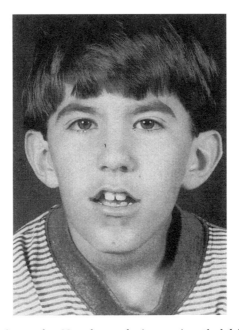

Patient at age 8 years and 6 months. Note hypotelorism, epicanthal folds, large ears, and dimpling below lower lip. (From Lewanda et al., 1995. *Am. J. Med. Genet.* 59:193–198. Copyright © 1995 John Wiley & Sons, Inc. Reprinted by permission of Wiley-Liss, Inc.)

REFERENCES

Gangarossa S, Mattina T, Romano V, Milana G, Mollica F, Schiliro G. 1996. Micromegakaryocytes in a patient with partial deletion of the long arm of chromosome 11[del(11)(q24.2qter)] and chronic thrombocytopenic purpura. *Am. J. Med. Genet.* 62:120–123.

Hertz JM, Tommerup N, Sorensen FB, Henriques UV, Nielsen A, Therkelsen AJ. 1995. Partial deletion 11q: report of a case with a large terminal deletion 11q21-qter without loss of telomeric sequences, and review of the literature. *Clin. Genet.* 47:231–235.

Lewanda AF, Morsey S, Reid CS, Jabs EW. 1995. Two craniosynostotic patients with 11q deletions, and review of 48 cases. *Am. J. Med. Genet.* 59:193–198.

Lin JH, Hou JW, Teng RJ, Tien HF, Lin KH. 1998. Jacobsen distal 11q deletion syndrome with a myelodysplastic change of hemopoietic cells. *Am. J. Med. Genet.* 75:341–344.

Obregon MG, Mingarelli R, Digilio MC, Zelante L, Giannotti A, Sabatino G, Dallapiccola B. 1992. Deletion 11q23 → qter (Jacobsen syndrome). Report of three new patients. *Ann. Genet.* 35(4):208–212.

Penny LA, Dell'Aquila M, Jones MC, Bergoffen J, Cunniff C, Fryns JP, Grace E, Graham JM Jr, Kousseff B, Mattina T, et al. 1995. Clinical and molecular characterization of patients with distal 11q deletions. *Am. J. Hum. Genet.* 56:676–683.

Pivnick EK, Velagaleti GV, Wilroy RS, Smith ME, Rose SR, Tipton RE, Tharapel AT. 1996. Jacobsen syndrome: report of a patient with severe eye anomalies, growth hormone deficiency, and hypothyroidism associated with deletion 11(q23q25) and review of 52 cases. *J. Med. Genet.* 33:772–778.

Stratton RF, Lazarus KH, Ritchie EJ, Bell AM. 1994. Deletion (11)(q14.1q21). *Am. J. Med. Genet.* 49:294–298.

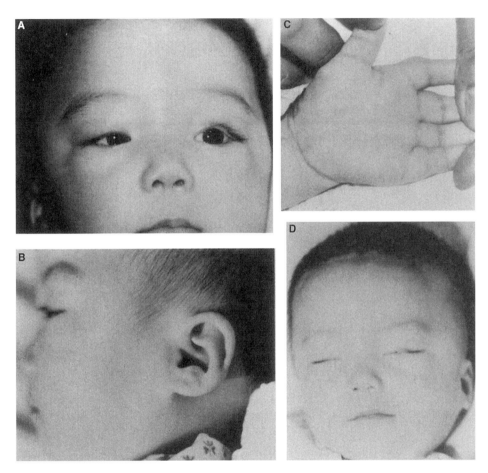

Note bilateral ptosis, abnormal eyelash arrangement (absence of eyelashes in inner one-third portion), small carp-shaped mouth (A), low-set and deformed ears (B), simian crease (C), and trigonocephaly and micrognathia (D). (From Lin et al., 1998. *Am. J. Med. Genet.* 75:341–344. Copyright © 1998 John Wiley & Sons, Inc. Reprinted by permission of Wiley-Liss, Inc.)

RING CHROMOSOME 11

Ring chromosome 11 is a very rare cytogenetic abnormality. Some researchers have proposed that this defect results in some features similar to del(11q). Due to the limited sample size, the characterization of a syndrome is not possible.

MAIN FEATURES: Growth retardation, microcephaly, psychomotor retardation

ABNORMALITIES

Growth: Growth retardation

Performance: Psychomotor retardation, developmental delay

Craniofacies: Microcephaly

Other: High and narrow palate, cafe-au-lait spots

OCCASIONAL ABNORMALITIES: Low nasal root, low-set ears, abnormal muscle tone

CLINICAL COURSE: Death in infancy is uncommon. Survival into adulthood is documented.

CYTOGENETICS: In almost all cases the defects are de novo.

REFERENCES

Fagan K, Suthers GK, Hardacre G. 1988. Ring chromosome 11 and cafe-au-lait spots. *Am. J. Med. Genet.* 30:911–916.

Niikawa N, Jinno Y, Tomiyasu T, Fukushima Y, Kudo K. 1981. Ring chromosome 11[46,XX,r(11)(p15q25)] associated with clinical features of the 11q- syndrome. *Ann. Genet.* 24(3):172–175.

Palka G, Verrotti A, Peca S, Mosca L, Lombardo G, Verrotti M, Morgese G. 1986. Ring chromosome 11: a case report and review of the literature. *Ann. Genet.* 29:55–58.

Romain DR, Gebbie OB, Parfitt RG, Columbano-Green LM, Smythe RH, Chapman CJ, Kerr A. 1983. Two cases of ring chromosome 11. *J. Med. Genet.* 20:380–382.

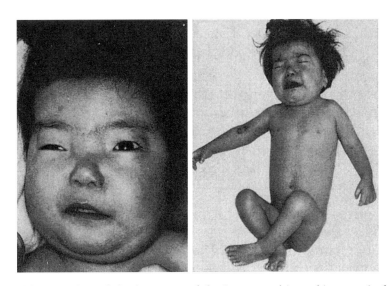

Note the frontal bossing, lateral displacement of the inner canthi, strabismus, pinched nose, and microretrognathia. (From Niikawa et al., 1981. *Ann. Genet.* 24:172–175. Reprinted with permission from Expansion Scientifique Francaise.)

CHROMOSOME 12p PARTIAL TRISOMY

Partial trisomy 12p is known to result in mental retardation and craniofacial dysmorphism. This defect can be de novo or result from parental chromosomal rearrangements. At least 33 cases have been described.

MAIN FEATURES: Mental retardation, short nose, everted lower lip.

ABNORMALITIES

Performance: Mental retardation, developmental delay, hypotonia

Craniofacies: High forehead, flat, round face, prominent cheeks, broad, flat nasal bridge, short nose, anteverted nostrils, long philtrum, wide mouth, everted lower lip, thin upper vermillion, malformed ears

Limbs: Foot deformities

Other: Congenital heart defects, short neck

OCCASIONAL ABNORMALITIES: Turricephaly, downward or upward slanted palpebral fissures and epicanthal folds

CLINICAL COURSE: Death in infancy is uncommon. Life expectancy is unknown

CYTOGENETICS: Most cases are familial, but de novo cases have been reported.

REFERENCES

Allen TL, Brothman AR, Carey JC, Chance PF. 1996. Cytogenetic and molecular analysis in trisomy 12p. *Am. J. Med. Genet.* 63:250–256.

Back E, Kratzer W, Zeitler S, Schempp W. 1997. De novo duplication of 12pter → p12.1: clinical and cytogenetic diagnosis confirmed by chromosome painting. *Clin. Genet.* 51:205–210.

Chen CP, Lin CC, Chuang CY, Lee CC, Chen WL, Jan SW, Lin SP. 1997. Prenatal diagnosis of partial trisomy 12 and partial trisomy 21 due to a 3:1 segregation of maternal reciprocal translocation t(12;21)(p13.3;q21). *Prenat. Diagn.* 17:675–680.

el-Shanti H, Khasawneh M, Hulsberg D, Major H, Patil S. 1997. A rare case of a liveborn with free, de novo, and partial trisomy 12 and an unusual phenotype. *Ann. Genet.* 40:175–180.

Guerrini R, Bureau M, Mattei MG, Battaglia A, Galland MC, Roger J. 1990. Trisomy 12p syndrome: a chromosomal disorder associated with generalized 3-Hz spike and wave discharges. *Epilepsia* 31:557–566.

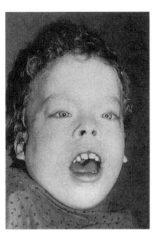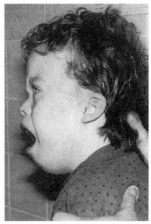

Patient at 5 years and 6 months. Note round face, prominent cheeks, high forehead, epicanthal folds, broad nasal bridge, short nose, anteverted nostrils, and large philtrum. (From Rauch et al., 1996. *Am. J. Med. Genet.* 63:243–249. Copyright © 1996 John Wiley & Sons, Inc. Reprinted by permission of Wiley-Liss, Inc.)

Rauch A, Trautmann U, Pfeiffer RA. 1996. Clinical and molecular cytogenetic observations in three cases of "trisomy 12p syndrome." *Am. J. Med. Genet.* 63:243–249.

Tayel S, McCorquodale MM, Rutherford T, Kurczynski TW, Abdel-Aziz AM, el-Gabaldy F, Sharaf EA. 1989. A case of de novo trisomy 12p syndrome. *Clin. Genet.* 35:382–386.

Zelante L, Calvano S, Dallapiccola B, Mingarelli R, Antonacci R, Chiovato L, Rocchi M. 1994. Patient with de novo 12p+ syndrome identified as dir dup (12)(p13) using subchromosomal painting libraries from somatic cell hybrids. *Clin. Genet.* 46:368–371.

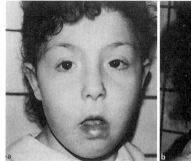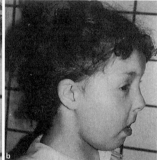

Note round face, high forehead, short palpebral fissures, telecanthus, strabismus, short nose, prominent nasal bridge, anteverted nostrils, long philtrum, and everted lower lip. (From Zelante et al., 1994. *Clin. Genet.* 46:368–371. Copyright © 1994 Munksgaard International Publishers Ltd., Copenhagen, Denmark, with permission.)

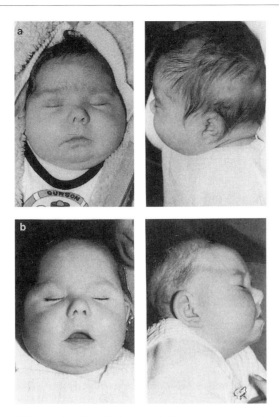

Patient at 6 weeks (a) and 9 months (b). Note round face, prominent cheeks, high forehead, epicanthal folds, broad nasal bridge, short nose, anteverted nostrils, and large philtrum. (From Rauch et al., 1996. *Am. J. Med. Genet.* 63:243–249. Copyright © 1996 John Wiley & Sons, Inc. Reprinted by permission of Wiley-Liss, Inc.)

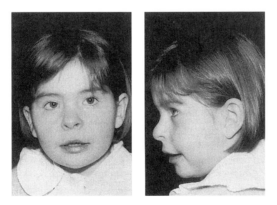

Patient at 4 years. Note round face, prominent cheeks, high forehead, short palpebral fissures, epicanthal folds, broad nasal bridge, short, upturned nose, anteverted nostrils, hypoplastic alae nasi, large philtrum, and thin lips. (From Rauch et al., 1996. *Am. J. Med. Genet.* 63:243–249. Copyright © 1996 John Wiley & Sons, Inc. Reprinted by permission of Wiley-Liss, Inc.)

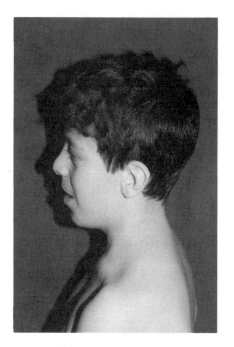

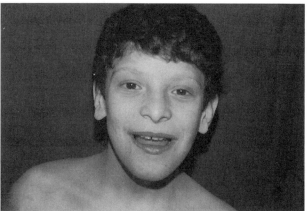

Patient at 12 years and 6 months. Note flat face, anteverted nares, wide philtrum, thick lower lip, and dysplastic ears. (From Kratzer et al., 1997. *Clin. Genet.* 51:205–210. Copyright © 1997 Munksgaard International Publishers Ltd., Copenhagen, Denmark, with permission.)

CHROMOSOME 12p TETRASOMY
Pallister–Killian Syndrome

In the mosaic form, this abnormality is also known as the Pallister–Killian syndrome. Pure 12p tetrasomy is very rare. The mosaic forms are thought to arise in post-zygotic stage of development. The percentage of tetrasomic cells do not correlate with the severity of the syndrome.

MAIN FEATURES: High birth weight, sparse scalp hair, high forehead, profound mental retardation.

ABNORMALITIES

Performance: Profound mental retardation, growth retardation, hypotonia, seizures

Craniofacies: Hypertelorism, alopecia, flat occiput, prognathism, prominent forehead, short neck with excess skin, low-set, malformed ears, short, wide nose, anteverted nares, high-arched palate, large, downturned mouth, long philtrum

Other: Absent speech, deafness, broad hands, short digits, shortened arm and leg bones, finger and nail anomalies, depigmented areas of skin, widely spaced nipples, undescended testes

In adulthood: Coarse and flat facial appearance, macroglossia, prognathism, everted lower lip, obesity, severe psychomotor retardation, hypertonia, contractures

OCCASIONAL ABNORMALITIES: Omphalocele, macroglossia, diaphragmatic hernia

CLINICAL COURSE: Many patients with 12p tetrasomy are stillborn or die in the neonatal period. Most survivors are non-ambulatory. The oldest reported patient is in his forties.

CYTOGENETICS: All cases arise de novo.

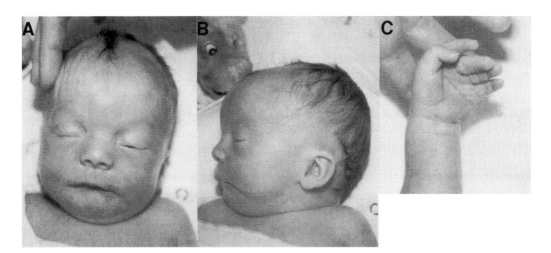

Patient as newborn showing (A) short palpebral fissures, short nose, simple philtrum, large mouth, short neck, (B) small mandible, low-set, dysplastic ears, alopecia of the forehead, (C) ulnar deviation of all fingers and simian crease. (From Horn et al., 1995. *J. Med. Genet.* 32:68–71. Reprinted with permission from BMJ Publishing Group.)

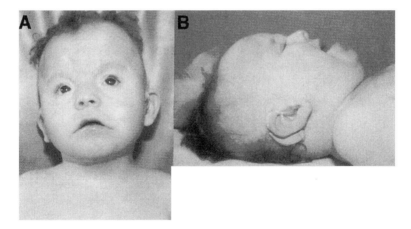

Patient at 1 year showing (A) high frontal hairline, prominent metopic suture, depigmentation over the right eyebrow, ptosis, hypertelorism, short nose with upturned nares, large mouth with downturned corners, and (B) temporofrontal alopecia and flat occiput. (From Horn et al., 1995. *J. Med. Genet.* 32:68–71. Reprinted with permission from BMJ Publishing Group.)

REFERENCES

Bergoffen J, Punnett H, Campbell TJ, Ross AJ 3rd, Ruchelli E, Zackai EH. 1993. Diaphragmatic hernia in tetrasomy 12p mosaicism. *J. Pediatr.* 122(4):603–606.

Horn D, Majewski F, Hildebrandt B, Korner H. 1995. Pallister–Killian syndrome: normal karyotype in prenatal chorionic villi, in postnatal lymphocytes, and in slowly growing epidermal cells, but mosaic tetrasomy 12p in skin fibroblasts. *J. Med. Genet.* 32:68–71.

Horneff G, Majewski F, Hildebrand B, Voit T, Lenard HG. 1993. Pallister–Killian syndrome in older children and adolescents. *Pediatr. Neurol.* 9(4):312–315.

Shivashankar L, Whitney E, Colmorgen G, Young T, Munshi G, Wilmoth D, Byrne K, Reeves G, Borgaonkar DS, Picciano SR, et al. 1988. Prenatal diagnosis of tetrasomy 47,XY,+i(12p) confirmed by in situ hybridization. *Prenat. Diagn.* 8:85–91.

Tejada MI, Uribarren A, Briones P, Vilaseca MA. 1992. A further prenatal diagnosis of mosaic tetrasomy 12p (Pallister–Killian syndrome). *Prenat. Diagn.* 12:529–534.

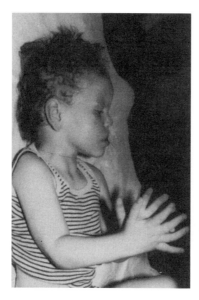 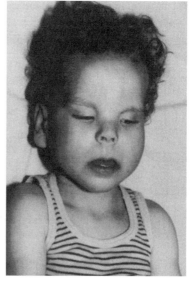

Patient at the age of 3 years and 4 months: high forehead with frontotemporal alopecia, short nose, enlarged tongue, broad mouth, and large ears. (From Horn et al., 1995. *J. Med. Genet.* 32:68–71. Reprinted with permission from BMJ Publishing Group.)

CHROMOSOME 12p PARTIAL MONOSOMY

Chromosome 12p partial deletion is a rare abnormality. Several features are common among most of the patients; however, these features are not unique to this chromosomal syndrome.

MAIN FEATURES: Brachydactyly, microcephaly, prominent nose, short stature

ABNORMALITIES

Growth: Postnatal growth failure

Performance: Mental retardation, hypotonia

Craniofacies: Microcephaly, narrow head, prominent occiput, long nose, broad nasal bridge, large, low-set ears, receding chin

Other: Brachydactyly, syndactyly of fingers 3 and 4, short stature

OCCASIONAL ABNORMALITIES: Congenital heart defects, cleft lip, genitourinary tract malformations

CLINICAL COURSE: Patients in their teens have been reported. Life into adulthood seems possible.

CYTOGENETICS: Most commonly de novo

REFERENCES

Bahring S, Nagai T, Toka HR, Nitz I, Toka O, Aydin A, Muhl A, Wienker TF, Schuster H, Luft FC. 1997. Deletion at 12p in a Japanese child with brachydactyly overlaps the assigned locus of brachydactyly with hypertension in a Turkish family. *Am. J. Hum. Genet.* 60:732–735.

Boilly-Dartigalongue B, Riviere D, Junien C, Couturier J, Toudic L, Marie F, Castel Y. 1985. [A new case of partial monosomy of chromosome 12,del(12)(p11.01 to p12.109) confirming the location of the gene for lactate dehydrogenase B]. *Ann. Genet.* 28:55–57.

Fryns JP, Kleczkowska A, Van den Berghe H. 1990. Interstitial deletion of the short arm of chromosome 12: report of a new patient and review of the literature. *Ann. Genet.* 33:43–45.

Hsu LY, Yu MT, Richkind KE, Van Dyke DL, Crandall BF, Saxe DF, Khodr GS, Mennuti M, Stetten G, Miller WA, Priest JH. 1996. Incidence and significance of chromosome mosaicism involving an autosomal structural abnormality diagnosed prenatally through amniocentesis: a collaborative study. *Prenat. Diagn.* 16:1–28.

Trautmann U, Pfeiffer RA. 1994. Interstitial deletion 12p13.1–13.3 in a mildly retarded infant with unilateral ectrodactyly. *Ann. Genet.* 37:147–149.

CHROMOSOME 12q PARTIAL TRISOMY

Chromosome 12q partial duplication is a clinically recognizable syndrome.

MAIN FEATURES: Excess nuchal skin, cryptorchidism, skeletal anomalies, sacral dimple

ABNORMALITIES

Performance: Developmental delay, mental retardation, psychomotor retardation, hypotonia

Craniofacies: Excess nuchal skin, short neck, micrognathia, brachycephaly, dolichocephaly, flat nasal bridge, wide mouth, low-set, malformed ears, high-arched palate, abnormal palpebral fissures

Other: Skeletal anomalies, bilateral transverse palmar creases, sacral dimple, genitourinary anomalies, bilateral cryptorchidism, wide-spaced nipples, digital malformations, hip subluxation, low posterior hairline

OCCASIONAL ABNORMALITIES: Eye abnormalities, short nose, flat-appearing face, seizures, brain anomalies

CLINICAL COURSE: Larger duplications of 12q have been lethal in infancy, while those with small distal duplications have survived into childhood.

CYTOGENETICS: Most patients result from a familial chromosomal translocation

REFERENCES

Dixon JW, Costa T, Teshima IE. 1993. Mosaicism for duplication 12q(12q13 → q24.2) in a dysmorphic male infant. *J. Med. Genet.* 30:70–72.

Jeziorowska A, Houck GE Jr, Yao XL, Sklower-Brooks SL, Wisniewski KE, Jenkins EC, Wisniewski HM. 1992. Reassessment of a chromosome 12q+ marker by fluorescent in situ hybridization (FISH). *Clin. Genet.* 42:124–128.

Koiffmann CP, Gonzalez CH, Vianna-Morgante AM, Kim CA, Odone-Filho V, Wajntal A. 1995. Neuroblastoma in a boy with MCA/MR syndrome, deletion 11q, and duplication 12q. *Am. J. Med. Genet.* 58:46–49.

Pratt NR, Bulugahapitiya DT. 1983. Partial trisomy 12q: a clinically recognisable syndrome. Genetic risks associated with translocations of chromosome 12q. *J. Med. Genet.* 20:86–89.

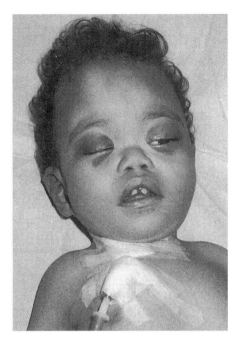

Note prominent forehead, epicanthus, flat nasal bridge, short bulbous nose, and exophthalmia. (From Koiffmann et al., 1995. *Am. J. Med. Genet.* 58:46–49. Copyright © 1995 John Wiley & Sons, Inc. Reprinted by permission of Wiley-Liss, Inc.)

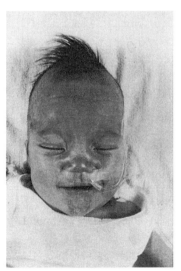 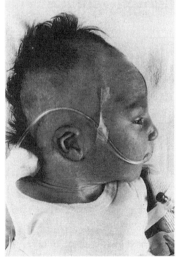 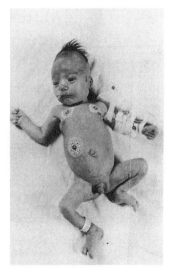

Patient at 5 days of age. Facial view (A). Note upward-slanting palpebral fissures, hypertelorism, broad, flat nasal bridge, and downturned mouth. Lateral view of face (B). Note low-set ears with abnormal helical folding and flattened occiput and forehead. Whole body (C). Note clenched hands and toes, widely spaced nipples, and shawl scrotum. Toes 1 and 2 are widespread. (From Dixon et al., 1993. *J. Med. Genet.* 30:70–72. Reprinted with permission from BMJ Publishing Group.)

CHROMOSOME 12q PARTIAL MONOSOMY

Chromosome 12q partial deletion is a very rare chromosome abnormality. One patient (Tonoki et al.) has features similar to Noonan's syndrome, but without a cardiac defect. The three patients described have only a few features in common.

MAIN FEATURES: Ear abnormalities, congenital heart defects, cleft lip/palate

ABNORMALITIES

Growth: Prenatal and postnatal growth retardation

Performance: Mental retardation

Eye: Hypertelorism

Craniofacies: Ear malformations, microretrognathia, cleft lip/palate

Other: Congenital heart defects

CLINICAL COURSE: Death in infancy is common.

CYTOGENETICS: Patients result from de novo defects and familial chromosomal translocations.

REFERENCES

Khan JY, Moss C, Roper HP. 1995. Aplasia cutis congenita with chromosome 12q abnormality. *Arch. Dis. Fetal. Neonatal. Ed.* 72:F205–F206.

Meinecke P, Meinecke R. 1987. Multiple malformation syndrome including cleft lip and palate and cardiac abnormalities due to an interstitial deletion of chromosome 12q. *J. Med. Genet.* 24:187.

Tonoki H, Saitoh S, Kobayashi K. 1998. Patient with del(12)(q12q13.12) manifesting abnormalities compatible with Noonan syndrome. *Am. J. Med. Genet.* 75:416–418.

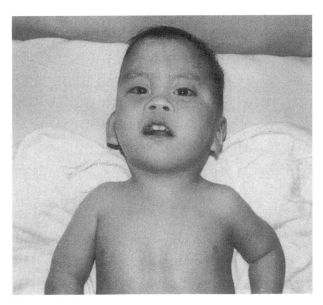

Patient at age 2 years. Note bilateral ptosis, strabismus, downward-slanting palpebral fissures, epicanthus, short nose with anteverted nares, long philtrum, and large, low-set ears. (From Tonoki et al., 1998. *Am. J. Med. Genet.* 75:416–418. Copyright © 1998 John Wiley & Sons, Inc. Reprinted by permission of Wiley-Liss, Inc.)

RING CHROMOSOME 12

Genotype–phenotype correlation is difficult to establish with ring chromosome abnormalities because of the large variation in clinical findings in these patients. This variation is due largely to the different breakpoints leading to the ring formation and to ring instability.

MAIN FEATURES: Severe growth retardation, mild mental retardation, café-au-lait spots.

ABNORMALITIES

Growth: Growth retardation

Performance: Mental retardation, speech deficiency

Craniofacies: Epicanthal folds, low-set ears, high-arched palate, microcephaly

Other: Multiple café-au-lait spots, clinodactyly of fifth finger, short stature

CLINICAL COURSE: The age range of the reported patients is between 13 months and 30 years.

CYTOGENETICS: All reported cases are de novo.

REFERENCES

Hajianpour MJ, Hajianpour AK, Habibian R, Wohlmuth C. 1996. Leiomyoma of uterus in a patient with ring chromosome 12: case presentation and literature review. *Am. J. Med. Genet.* 63:335–339.

Park JP, Graham JM Jr, Andrews PA, Wurster-Hill DH. 1988. Ring chromosome 12. *Am. J. Med. Genet.* 29:437–440.

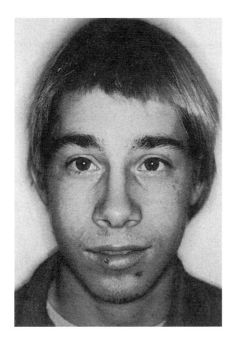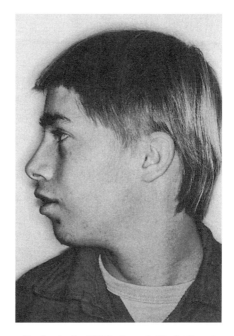

AP and lateral view of the patient at 19 years. (From Park et al., 1988. *Am. J. Med. Genet.* 29:437–440. Copyright © 1988 John Wiley & Sons, Inc. Reprinted by permission of Wiley-Liss, Inc.)

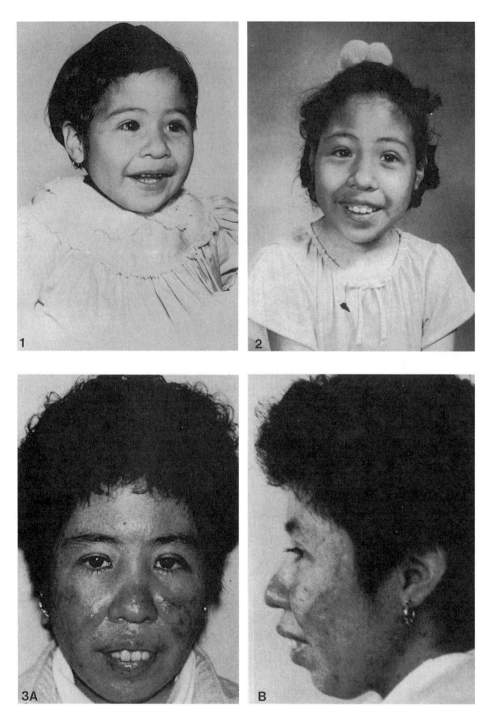

Patient at 3 years (1). Patient at 12 years (2). Patient at 30 years (3A,B). Note epicanthic folds, long eyelashes, broad nasal bridge, and micrognathia with overbite. (From Hajianpour et al., 1996. *Am. J. Med. Genet.* 63:335–339. Copyright © 1996 John Wiley & Sons, Inc. Reprinted by permission of Wiley-Liss, Inc.)

CHROMOSOME 13 TRISOMY
Patau Syndrome

Described by Patau et al. in 1960, this syndrome is readily recognizable because of its characteristic pattern of craniofacial and limb malformations.

MAIN FEATURES: Microphthalmia, cleft lip and palate, polydactyly, scalp ulcers

GENERAL CHARACTERISTICS: Most newborns and fetuses with trisomy 13 have normal prenatal growth pattern with the average birth weight being slightly below normal. Microcephaly disproportionate to length is common. The severity or extent of the defects can vary a great deal. Congenital heart defects are present in 50% of the cases. Though septal defects are common, any type of cardiac malformation can be associated with trisomy 13. An increased frequency of nuclear projections in circulating polymorphonuclear leukocytes is a unique hematological manifestation of trisomy 13. (Also see triploidy). Persistence of higher than normal level of fetal hemoglobin is also common.

ABNORMALITIES

Craniofacies: Cleft lip and palate, microphthalmia, nevus flammeus over the forehead, nose, and upper lip, scalp defects with mild to moderate malformation of the pinnae

Limbs: Postaxial polydactyly typically may involve any or all limbs, camptodactyly, overlapping digits, hyperconvex nails, transverse palmar creases, prominence of the heels is more common than rocker-bottom feet

Genitourinary: Hypospadias and cryptorchidism in the male, hypoplastic ovaries in the female, horseshoe kidneys, renal cysts, and hydronephrosis in either sex

Other: Central nervous system (CNS) malformation usually including the midline structures, holoprosencephaly, agenesis of the corpus callosum, fused thalami, cyclopia

CLINICAL COURSE: Most infants born with trisomy 13 succumb during the first few weeks of life primarily due to central apnea. Survival to 1 year may be seen in 5–10% of the cases. Growth and mental retardation are severe to profound without exception. The rare adults with trisomy 13 show profound mental retardation.

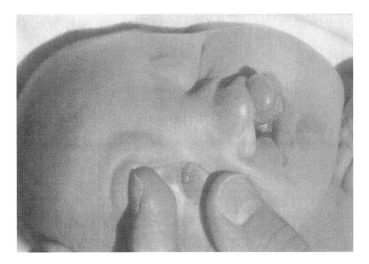

Newborn with trisomy 13 showing severe bilateral microphthalmia, broad nasal bridge, and bilateral cleft lip and palate.

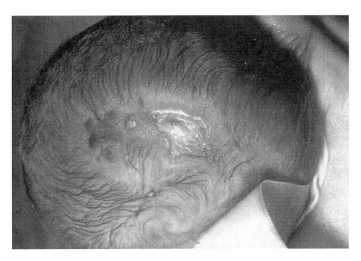

Scalp defects in a newborn with trisomy 13.

CYTOGENETICS: Most cases of trisomy 13 are complete trisomies resulting from nondisjunctional errors. Maternal-age effect is known but not as pronounced as in trisomy 21. At least 10% of the cases involve structural aberrations such as translocations and inversions. Partial trisomy 13 can occur secondary to malsegregation of parental balanced translocations, inversions, or complex multichromosomal rearrangements. Phenotype–karyotype correlation studies have allowed phenotype mapping of chromosome 13q and have identified features more or less unique to the proximal and distal halves of 13q.

CHROMOSOME 13 PARTIAL TRISOMY: Partial trisomy 13 can be separated into two distinctive syndromes: the proximal trisomy 13q involving bands 13q11q22 triplication and distal trisomy 13q primarily attributed to bands 13q32-qter.

Proximal trisomy 13q is characterized by craniofacial anomalies, including depressed nasal bridge, stubby nose, cleft lip and palate, increased nuclear projections in neutrophils, and persistence of high fetal hemoglobin levels beyond the first few weeks of life. Moderate to severe mental deficiency is present but survival is prolonged as compared to full trisomy. Clinical recognition of this syndrome is not possible due to the relatively nonspecific findings.

Distal trisomy 13 is more common and has more of the features associated with full trisomy 13. These features include facial midline hemangiomas, postaxial polydactyly, transverse palmer crease, palatal and genitourinary abnormalities. Growth and mental retardation tend to be severe.

Interestingly neither syndrome is associated with some of the more severe trisomy 13 malformations such as severe microphthalmia, anophthalmia, holoprosencaphaly, and scalp defects.

REFERENCES

Baty BJ, Blackburn BL, Carey JC. 1994. Natural history of trisomy 18 and trisomy 13: I. Growth, physical assessment, medical histories, survival, and recurrence risk. *Am. J. Med. Genet.* 49:175–188.

Baty BJ, Jorde LB, Blackburn BL, Carey JC. 1994. Natural history of trisomy 18 and trisomy 13: II. Psychomotor development. *Am. J. Med. Genet.* 49:189–194.

Bonioli E, Crisalli M, Monteverde R, Vianello MG. 1981. Karyotype-phenotype correlation in partial trisomy 13: report of a case due to maternal translocation. *Am. J. Dis. Child.* 135:1115–1117.

Chen CP, Liu FF, Jan SW, Su TH, Lan CC. 1996. A concealed penis mimicking penile agenesis in an infant with trisomy 13. *Clin. Genet.* 50:156–158.

Gilgenkrantz S, Defeche C, Stehlin S, Gregoire MJ. 1981. Proximal trisomy 13: a family with balanced reciprocal translocation t(8;13) in seven members and Robertsonian translocation t(13;14) in three members. *Hum. Genet.* 58:436–440.

Hook EB. 1980. Rates of 47, +13 and 46 translocation D/13 Patau syndrome in live births and comparison with rates in fetal deaths and at amniocentesis. *Am. J. Hum. Genet.* 32:849–858.

Lehman CD, Nyberg DA, Winter TC 3rd, Kapur RP, Resta RG, Luthy DA. 1995. Trisomy 13 syndrome: prenatal US findings in a review of 33 cases. *Radiology* 194:217–222.

Moerman P, Fryns JP, van der Steen K, Kleczkowska A, Lauweryns J. 1988. The pathology of trisomy 13 syndrome: a study of 12 cases. *Hum. Genet.* 80:349–356.

Patau K, Smith DW, Therman E, Inhorn SL, Wagner HP. 1960. Multiple congenital anomaly caused by extra autosome. *Lancet* I:790–793.

Rodriguez JI, Garcia M, Morales C, Morillo A, Delicado A. 1990. Trisomy 13 syndrome and neural tube defects. *Am. J. Med. Genet.* 36:513–516.

Tharapel SA, Lewandowski RC, Tharapel AT, Wilroy RS Jr. 1986. Phenotype-karyotype correlation in patients trisomic for various segments of chromosome 13. *J. Med. Genet.* 23:310–315.

Zoll B, Wolf J, Lensing-Hebben D, Pruggmayer M, Thorpe B. 1993. Trisomy 13 (Patau syndrome) with an 11-year survival. *Clin. Genet.* 43:46–50.

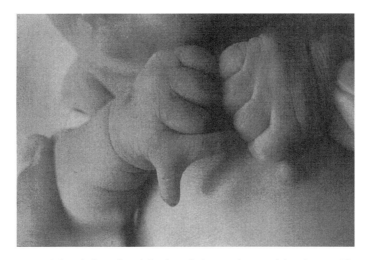

Postaxial polydactyly of the hands in newborn with trisomy 13.

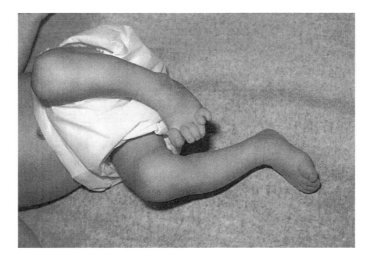

Boy with distal trisomy 13q with less severe malformations. Note unilateral postaxial polydactyly of the foot.

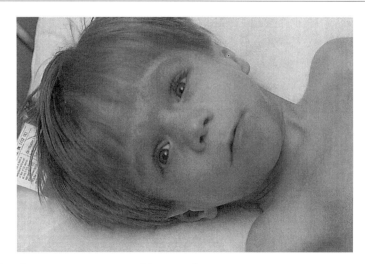

Patient with distal trisomy 13q. Note mild nevus flammeus over the glabella and forehead and absence of cleft lip and microphthalmia.

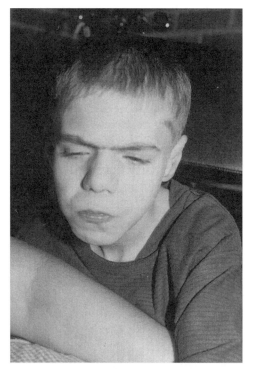

Same patient as (Figures 4 and 5) a teenager with profound mental retardation.

CHROMOSOME 13q PARTIAL MONOSOMY

Monosomy 13q may result from terminal or interstitial deletions or ring formation. Many malformations are associated with 13q deletion.

MAIN FEATURES: Growth deficiency, mental retardation, microcephaly, thumb hypoplasia

ABNORMALITIES

Performance: Mental retardation is severe and always present

Craniofacies: Microcephaly, large forehead, low-set ears, hypertelorism, downward-slanted palpebral fissures, blepharophimosis, microphthalmia, microcornea and iris coloboma, protruding premaxilla, micrognathia, highly arched palate, and pterygium colli

Limbs: Hypoplasia of the digits, particularly of the thumbs, fourth and fifth toe syndactyly, missing fifth toes, subluxation of the hips, and clubfoot

Genitourinary: List circled entries under this subheading

Other: Organ system malformations have included cardiac defects—primarily septal defects and patent ductus arteriosus. Agenesis of the corpus callosum, adrenal hypoplasia, agenesis or hypoplasia of the kidneys, hypoplasia of the genitals, ureteral anomalies, bifid scrotum and hypospadias leading to an ambiguous external genital anatomy.

OCCASIONAL ABNORMALITIES: Neural tube defects, Hirschsprung's disease, intestinal atresia, Waardenburg syndrome, Moebius syndrome. Retinoblastoma may be associated with deletions that involve band 13q14

CLINICAL COURSE: High mortality during infancy. Survival to adulthood has been documented in patients with this syndrome.

CYTOGENETICS: Most cases are de novo deletions involving variable 13q segments. Small interstitial deletions and familial chromosomal translocations are also known.

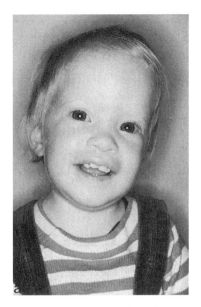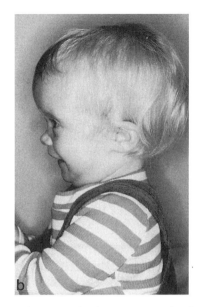

Frontal (a) and lateral (b) views of the face at age 2, depicting high, prominent forehead, frontal bossing, and low-set, malformed pinnae. (From Tranebjaerg et al., 1988. *Am. J. Med. Genet.* 29:739–753. Copyright © 1988 John Wiley & Sons, Inc. Reprinted by permission of Wiley-Liss, Inc.)

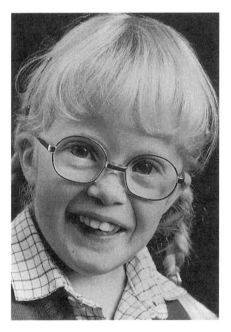

Patient shown above at 6 years. (From Tranebjaerg et al., 1988. *Am. J. Med. Genet.* 29:739–753. Copyright © 1988 John Wiley & Sons, Inc. Reprinted by permission of Wiley-Liss, Inc.)

REFERENCES

Allderdice PW, Davis JG, Miller OJ, Klinger HP, Warburton D, Miller DA, Allen FH Jr, Abrams CAL, McGilvray E. 1969. The 13q del syndrome. *Am. J. Hum. Genet.* 21:499–512.

Brown S, Gersen S, Anyane-Yeboa K, Warburton D. 1993. Preliminary definition of a "critical region" of chromosome 13 in q32: report of 14 cases with 13q deletions and review of the literature. *Am. J. Med. Genet.* 45:52–59.

Chen CP, Liu FF, Jan SW, Wang KG, Lan CC. 1996. Prenatal diagnosis of partial monosomy 13q associated with occipital encephalocoele in a fetus. *Prenat. Diagn.* 16:664–666.

Dean JC, Simpson S, Couzin DA, Stephen GS. 1991. Interstitial deletion of chromosome 13: prognosis and adult phenotype. *J. Med. Genet.* 28:533–535.

Emanuel BS, Zackai EH, Moreau L, Coates P, Orrechio E. 1979. Interstitial deletion 13q33 resulting from maternal insertional translocation. *Clin. Genet.* 16:340–346.

Lamont MA, Fitchett M, Dennis NR. 1989. Interstitial deletion of distal 13q associated with Hirschsprung's disease. *J. Med. Genet.* 26:100–104.

Nichols WW, Miller RC, Hoffman E, Albert D, Weichselbaum RR, Nove J, Little JB. 1979. Interstitial deletion of chromosome 13 and associated congenital anomalies. *Hum. Genet.* 52:169–173.

Noel B, Quack B, Rethore MO. 1976. Partial deletions and trisomies of chromosome 13; mapping of bands associated with particular malformations. *Clin. Genet.* 9:593–602.

Talvik I, Ounap K, Bartsch O, Ilus T, Uibo O, Talvik T. 2000. Boy with celiac disease, malformations, and ring chromosome 13 with deletion 13q32 → qter. *Am. J. Med. Genet.* 93:399–402.

Tranebjaerg L, Nielsen KB, Tommerup N, Warburg M, Mickkelsen M. 1988. Interstitial deletion 13q: further delineation of the syndrome by clinical and high-resolution chromosome analysis of five patients. *Am. J. Med. Genet.* 29:739–753.

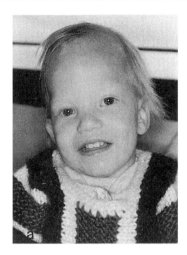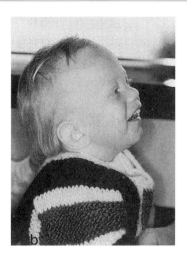

Front (a) and side view (b) of the face of 2-year-old girl showing remarkable similarity to previous patient with long, oval-shaped face, prominent, tall forehead, and large low-set ears. (From Tranebjaerg et al., 1988. *Am. J. Med. Genet.* 29:739–753. Copyright © 1988 John Wiley & Sons, Inc. Reprinted by permission of Wiley-Liss, Inc.)

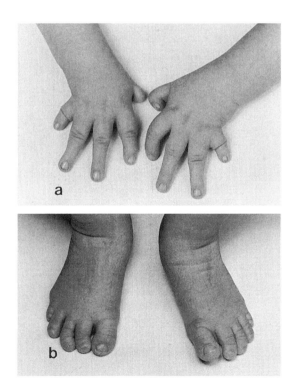

Hands (a) and feet (b) of patient at age 3 years and 6 months. Hands show shortening of the thumbs and fifth fingers. Radiographs showed absent left first metacarpal and fusion of the fourth and fifth metacarpals bilaterally. (From Tranebjaerg et al., 1988. *Am. J. Med. Genet.* 29:739–753. Copyright © 1988 John Wiley & Sons, Inc. Reprinted by permission of Wiley-Liss, Inc.)

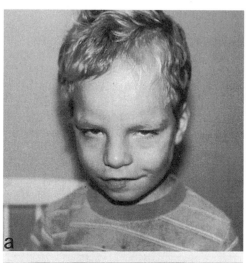
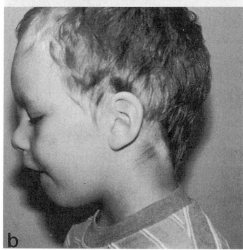

Frontal (a) and lateral (b) views of patient at age 6 years. Note prominent forehead, micrognathia, and broad nasal root. (From Tranebjaerg et al., 1988. *Am. J. Med. Genet.* 29:739–753. Copyright © 1988 John Wiley & Sons, Inc. Reprinted by permission of Wiley-Liss, Inc.)

CHROMOSOME 14 TRISOMY MOSAICISM

Trisomy for the entire chromosome14 appears to be compatible with live birth only in the presence of a normal cell line. The first case was described by Murker et al. in 1970. Since then at least 15 live-born and four prenatal cases have been described.

MAIN FEATURES: Growth and psychomotor retardation, facial asymmetry wide mouth

GENERAL CHARACTERISTICS: The syndrome has a variable phenotype due to the presence of mosaicism. Live-born infants have shown poor growth, severe psychomotor retardation, craniofacial, cardiac, central nervous system, limb, and cutaneous pigmentary abnormalities.

ABNORMALITIES

Craniofacies: Microcephaly, prominent forehead, micrognathia, facial asymmetry, low-set, dysplastic ears, deeply set, small eyes, upward- or downward-slanting palpebral fissures, broad nasal bridge, wide mouth, thick lips, cleft palate and cleft lip

Limbs: Asymmetric limbs, hip dislocation, hand contractures, and rocker-bottom feet

Other: Tetralogy of Fallot, atrial septal defect, cryptorchidism, small penis, and renal insufficiency may be present. Alobar holoprosencephaly was found in a fetus. Another fetus was found to be growth restricted without any malformation detectable by sonography. Nuclear projections of neutrophils similar to those found in trisomy 13 and triploidy have been reported.

CLINICAL COURSE: Most reported cases are children. Probability of survival to adulthood unknown.

CYTOGENETICS: Free trisomy 14 of maternal as well as paternal origin has been found. Dissociation of a t(14q15q) and dicentric chromosome 14 have been reported. The frequency of cells trisomic for chromosome 14 has varied greatly in different tissues of the same patient and among different patients. An apparent lack of correlation between cytogenetic findings in amniotic fluid and the severity of the fetal phenotype has pointed out the difficulty in counseling families regarding the expected outcome. There has been no parental-age effect or imprinting effect noted.

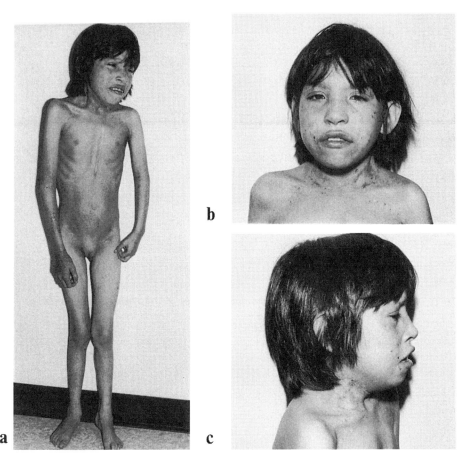

Seven-year-old girl with trisomy 14 in 41% of peripheral blood lymphocytes showing short stature, poor weight gain, short, wide neck, upward-slanting palpebral fissures, mild ptosis, large ears, broad nasal root, wide mouth, and thick lips. (From Johnson et al., 1979. *Am. J. Med. Genet.* 3:331–339. Copyright © 1979 John Wiley & Sons, Inc. Reprinted by permission of Wiley-Liss, Inc.)

REFERENCES

Cheung SW, Kolacki PL, Watson MS, Crane JP. 1988. Prenatal diagnosis, fetal pathology, and cytogenetic analysis of mosaic trisomy 14. *Prenat. Diagn.* 8:677–682.

Dallapiccola B, Ferranti G, Giannotti A, Novelli G, Pasquini L, Porfirio B. 1984. A live infant with trisomy 14 mosaicism and nuclear abnormalities of the neutrophils. *J. Med. Genet.* 21:467–470.

del Mazo J, Abrisqueta JA. 1984. Trisomy 14 by paternal origin. *Hum. Genet.* 68:193.

Fujimoto A, Lin MS, Korula SR, Wilson MG. 1985. Trisomy 14 mosaicism with t(14;15)(q11;p11) in offspring of a balanced translocation carrier mother. *Am. J. Med. Genet.* 22:333–342.

Johnson VP, Aceto T Jr, Likness C. 1979. Trisomy 14 mosaicism: case report and review. *Am. J. Med. Genet.* 3:331–339.

Kaplan LC, Wayne A, Crowell S, Latt SA. 1986. Trisomy 14 mosaicism in a liveborn male: clinical report and review of the literature. *Am. J. Med. Genet.* 23:925–930.

Keitges EA, Skogerbor KJ, Luthardt FW. 1993. Mosaic trisomy 14 diagnosed at amniocentesis, confirmed in CVS cultures, but absent in fetal skin cultures. *Cytogenet. Cell Genet.* 63:251.

Lambert I, Kemp J, Jackson J, Joyce H, Mann S, Kan A, Smith A. 1994. Prenatal diagnosis and post-mortem study of a fetus with mosaic trisomy 14 due to a dic(14)(p11). *Prenat. Diagn.* 14:507–510.

Sepulveda W, Monckeberg MJ, Be C. 1998. Twin pregnancy discordant for trisomy 14 mosaicism: prenatal sonographic findings. *Prenat. Diagn.* 18:481–484.

Wegner RD, Hohle R, Karkut G, Sperling K. 1988. Trisomy 14 mosaicism leading to cytogenetic discrepancies in chorionic villi sampled at different times. *Prenat. Diagn.* 8:239–243.

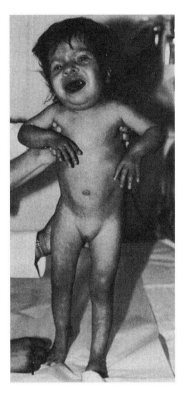

Two-year-old girl with 46,XX/46,XX,der t(14;15)(p11;q11)mat. The abnormal cell line was found in 56% of her lymphocytes and 100% of the fibroblasts. Note pigmentary abnormalities of the skin, poor growth, and body asymmetry. Note similarity of facial anomalies to those of previous patient. (From Fujimoto et al., 1985. *Am. J. Med. Genet.* 22:333–342. Copyright © 1985 John Wiley & Sons, Inc. Reprinted by permission of Wiley-Liss, Inc.)

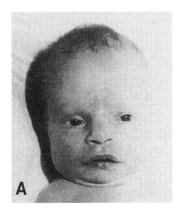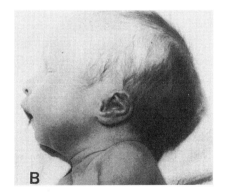

Facial close-up of one-week-old male showing prominent forehead, small palpebral fissures, broad nasal bridge, micrognathia, and short, low-set, posteriorly rotated ears. Twenty-five percent of the peripheral blood lymphocytes showed trisomy 14. (From Kaplan et al., 1986. *Am. J. Med. Genet.* 23:925–930. Copyright © 1986 John Wiley & Sons, Inc. Reprinted by permission of Wiley-Liss, Inc.)

CHROMOSOME 14q PARTIAL TRISOMY

Since the first description by Allderdice et al. in 1971, more than 50 cases with duplication of various segments of 14q have been described. A clinically recognizable syndrome has been difficult to define, perhaps due to complexities related to the presence of imprinted loci on 14q. The clinical findings are based on review of 35 published cases.

MAIN FEATURES: Microcephaly, micrognathia, microphthalmia, malformed pinnae.

GENERAL CHARACTERISTICS: Prenatal growth has been normal with few exceptions. However, postnatal growth and moderate to severe psychomotor retardation are usually present with a few notable exceptions (see below).

ABNORMALITIES

Craniofacies: Microcephaly is common. Sparse hair may be seen in infants. Facial anomalies also have varied from minimal nondescript dysmorphism to more severe anomalies such as choanal stenosis, microphthalmia, and iris coloboma in occasional patients. Malformed ears have been noted in at least 60% of the cases. Facial asymmetry may be present. The palpebral fissures have been upward-slanting or downward-slanting, nose has been variously described as bulbous, thin, or parrotlike. Micrognathia is very common. Downturned corners of the mouth and cleft of the secondary palate are also seen.

Genitourinary: Genital anomalies include cryptorchidism and hypospadias in about 30% of the males, and hypoplasia of the labia majora and fusion of the labia minora in females.

Limbs: Clubfoot, syndactyly, prominent finger tip pads, and joint contractures have been noted. There is no characteristic dermatoglyphic pattern associated with partial trisomy 14q.

Organs: Congenital heart defects, usually septal defects, are found in about 45% of the patients. Prenatally diagnosed cases have been found to have omphalocele.

Other: A father and daughter with apparently identical duplication of the 14q24.3q32 segment have been described with discordant phenotypes. Whereas the child had congenital anomalies, the father was phenotypically normal. The presence of maternally imprinted genes in the duplicated region was a possible explanation. Alternatively, the region may have silenced genes, not subject to dosage effect; thus, implying that duplication was unrelated to the phenotype.

Another interesting observation is a child reported by Lemire et al. (1997) whose phenotype evolved from Williams syndrome-like in infancy to Prader-Willi-like in later childhood. Both syndromes were excluded by appropriate studies.

Also, at least one instance of a child that meets diagnostic criteria for the Coloboma, Heart defect, Atresia choanae, Retardation, Genital anomalies, Ear anomalies (CHARGE) association has been found with duplication of bands 14q22q24.3.

CYTOGENETICS: Partial trisomy 14 has resulted from malsegregation of reciprocal translocations involving various autosomes. Recombinants secondary to pericentric inversion and de novo inverted and tandem duplications have also been reported. Paternal as well as maternal transmissions have been documented. Duplications of the 14q23 or q24 band seem to be most consistently associated with many of the craniofacial malformations described above. No distinctive syndrome due to duplication of the more proximal segments has evolved.

REFERENCES

Allderdice PW, Miller OJ, Miller DA, Breg WR, Gendel E, Zelson C. 1971. Familial translocation involving chromosomes 6, 14 and 20, identified by quinacrine fluorescence. *Humangenetik*. 13:205–209.

Carr DM, Jones-Quartey K, Vartanian MV, Moore-Kaplan H. 1987. Duplication 14(q31 → qter). *J. Med. Genet.* 24:372–374.

Duckett DP, Roberts E, McKeever P, Young ID. 1990. Prenatal diagnosis of trisomy for the distal two-thirds of the long arm of chromosome 14(q21 → qter). *Prenat. Diagn.* 10:261–264.

Gilgenkrantz S, Vigneron J, Peter MO, Dufier JL, Teboul M, Chery M, Keyeux G, Lefranc MP. 1990. Distal trisomy 14q. I. Clinical and cytogenetical studies. *Hum. Genet.* 85:612–616.

Lemire EG, Cardwell S. 1999. Unusual phenotype in partial trisomy 14. *Am. J. Med. Genet.* 87:294–296.

Mignon-Ravix C, Mugneret F, Stavropoulou C, Depetris D, Van Kien PK, Mattei MG. 2001. Maternally inherited duplication of the possible imprinted 14q31 region. *J. Med. Genet.* 38:343–347.

North KN, Wu BL, Cao BN, Whiteman DA, Korf BR. 1995. CHARGE association in a child with de novo inverted duplication (14)(q22 → q24.3). *Am. J. Med. Genet.* 57:610–614.

Pot ML, Giltay JC, van Wilsen A, Breslau-Siderius EJ. 1996. Unbalanced karyotype, dup 14(q13–q22), in a mother and her two children. *Clin. Genet.* 50:398–402.

Robin NH, Harari-Shacham A, Schwartz S, Wolff DJ. 1997. Duplication 14(q24.3q31) in a father and daughter: delineation of a possible imprinted region. *Am. J. Med. Genet.* 71:361–365.

Strain JE, Smith AC, Ward BE, Robinson A. 1981. Inverted tandem duplication of the middle segment of the long arm of chromosome 14. *Pediatrics* 67:273–276.

Verma RS, Kleyman SM, Conte RA, Laqui-Pili C, Bennett H. 1998. Tandem duplication of chromosome 14(q12q13). *Ann. Genet.* 40:209–210.

CHROMOSOME 14q PARTIAL MONOSOMY

Deletion of the long arm of chromosome 14 is rarer than 14q duplications. Most patients have the deletion identified because of developmental delay and facial dysmorphism. Birth weight usually has been normal. Postnatal growth failure and global developmental delay are common, but varying in severity. This summary is based on review of a relatively small number of less than 20 published cases, excluding those with ring chromosome 14.

MAIN FEATURES: Deeply set eyes, chubby cheeks, prominent philtrum

ABNORMALITIES

Craniofacies: Microcephaly and flat occiput are consistent. The face may be round with full cheeks or elongated. The palate is high and rarely cleft. Bushy eyebrows, short stubby nose with an upturned broad tip, long upper lip with deeply marked philtrum, thin upper lip, and micrognathia are commonly found. The palpebral fissures are small and downward slanting in some cases.

Organs: Central nervous system malformations involving enlarged ventricles, thin corpus callosum, holoprosencephaly, cebocephaly, absent pituitary gland, anophthalmia, retinal dystrophy, and macular abnormality have been found in isolated cases. Atrial and ventricular septal defects have been found. Genital anomalies including hypospadias, cryptorchidism, horseshoe kidney, and hydronephrosis may be present.

CLINICAL COURSE: Mental retardation is present in all cases. The severity of cognitive impairment has varied. Most reported cases are fetuses or young children and there are no longitudinal follow-up studies at this time.

CYTOGENETICS: Most cases of 14q monosomy are due to interstitial deletion of bands 14q22, 14q23, 14q31, or 14q32. The smallest deletion was found by molecular studies of an apparently balanced inherited Robertsonian translocation t(14;21) in an infant with abnormal facial features, hypotonia, and developmental delay. Gonadal mosaicism has been suggested on at least two occasions. Thus a higher than average recurrence risk may exist for parents of apparently de novo cases. However, quantitative recurrence risk estimate is not available. There is insufficient information at this time to define distinctive proximal and distal 14q monosomy syndromes.

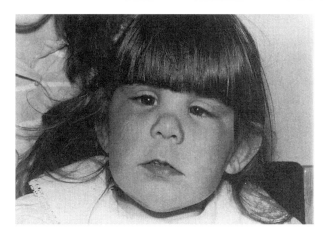

Facial features of a girl 3 years and 6 months of age with interstitial deletion of 14q24.3q32.1. Note epicanthal folds, short, upturned nose, long upper lip with deep philtrum, thin upper lip vermillion, and large, fleshy ears. (From Karnitis et al., 1992. *Am. J. Med. Genet.* 44:153–157. Copyright © 1992 John Wiley & Sons, Inc. Reprinted by permission of Wiley-Liss, Inc.)

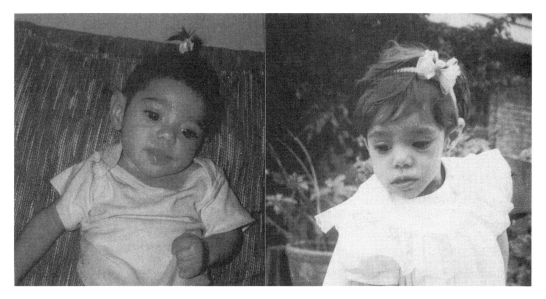

Infant with interstitial deletion of 14q11.2q21.1 at 6 months and 12 months. Patient had low birth weight, failure to thrive, microcephaly, relatively mild facial dysmorphism, and severe developmental delay. (From Shapira et al., 1994. *Am. J. Med. Genet.* 52:44–50. Copyright © 1994 John Wiley & Sons, Inc. Reprinted by permission of Wiley-Liss, Inc.)

REFERENCES

Bennett CP, Betts DR, Seller MJ. 1991. Deletion 14q(q22q23) associated with anophthalmia, absent pituitary, and other abnormalities. *J. Med. Genet.* 28:280–281.

Bonthron DT, Smith SJ, Fantes J, Gosden CM. 1993. De novo microdeletion on an inherited Robertsonian translocation chromosome: a cause for dysmorphism in the apparently balanced translocation carrier. *Am. J. Hum. Genet.* 53:629–637.

Bruyere H, Favre B, Douvier S, Nivelon-Chevalier A, Mugneret F. 1996. De novo interstitial proximal deletion of 14q and prenatal diagnosis of holoprosencephaly. *Prenat. Diagn.* 16:1059–1060.

Byth BC, Costa MT, Teshima IE, Wilson WG, Carter NP, Cox DW. 1995. Molecular analysis of three patients with interstitial deletions of chromosome band 14q31. *J. Med. Genet.* 32:564–567.

Chen CP, Lee CC, Chen LF, Chuang CY, Jan SW, Chen BF. 1997. Prenatal diagnosis of de novo proximal interstitial deletion of 14q associated with cebocephaly. *J. Med. Genet.* 34:777–778.

Devriendt K, Fryns JP, Chen CP. 1998. Holoprosencephaly in deletions of proximal chromosome 14q. *J. Med. Genet.* 35:612.

Elliott J, Maltby EL, Reynolds B. 1993. A case of deletion 14(q22.1 → q22.3) associated with anophthalmia and pituitary abnormalities. *J. Med. Genet.* 30:251–252.

Gorski JL, Uhlmann WR, Glover TW. 1990. A child with multiple congenital anomalies and karyotype 46,XY,del(14)(q31q32.3): further delineation of chromosome 14 interstitial deletion syndrome. *Am. J. Med. Genet.* 37:471–474.

Karnitis SA, Burns K, Sudduth KW, Golden WL, Wilson WG. 1992. Deletion (14)(q24.3q32.1): evidence for a distinct clinical phenotype. *Am. J. Med. Genet.* 44:153–157.

Lemyre E, Lemieux N, Decarie JC, Lambert M. 1998. Del(14)(q22.1q23.2) in a patient with anophthalmia and pituitary hypoplasia. *Am. J. Med. Genet.* 77:162–165.

Miller BA, Jayakar P, Capo H. 1992. Child with multiple congenital anomalies and mosaicism 46,XX/46,XX,del(14)(q32.3). *Am. J. Med. Genet.* 44:635–637.

Nielsen J, Homma A, Rasmussen K, Ried E, Sorensen K, Saldana-Garcia P. 1978. Deletion 14q and pericentric inversion 14. *J. Med. Genet.* 15:236–238.

Ortigas AP, Stein CK, Thomson LL, Hoo JJ. 1997. Delineation of 14q32.3 deletion syndrome. *J. Med. Genet.* 34:515–517.

Schuffenhauer S, Leifheit HJ, Lichtner P, Peters H, Murken J, Emmerich P. 1999. De novo deletion (14)(q11.2q13) including PAX9: clinical and molecular findings. *J. Med. Genet.* 36:233–236.

Shapira SK, Anderson KL, Orr-Urtregar A, Craigen WJ, Lupski JR, Shaffer LG. 1994. De novo proximal interstitial deletions of 14q: cytogenetic and molecular investigations. *Am J. Med. Genet.* 52:44–50.

UNIPARENTAL DISOMY 14

Engel (1980) proposed uniparental disomy (UPD), defined as the presence of two homologous chromosomes of one parent in a diploid individual, as a mechanism for human malformation. Maternal UPD (14) and paternal UPD (14) appear to be two distinctive syndromes as might be expected in the presence of differentially imprinted loci on the chromosome. This summary is based on a review of 24 published cases of UPD14.

MAIN FEATURES: Prenatal and postnatal growth retardation, variable developmental delay

GENERAL CHARACTERISTICS: Intrauterine and postnatal growth retardation appear to be consistent features present in all published cases. Whether bias of ascertainment plays a role is not known since most cases have been ascertained through phenotypically abnormal patients.

ABNORMALITIES

Craniofacies: These anomalies are mild in maternal UPD (14) cases. Macrocephaly, dolichocephaly, high-arched palate, hypoplasia of the scapha helix, and prominent nasal bridge have been noted. Infants may show excessively large fontanelle.

Limbs: Short hands and feet are always present.

Other: Precocious puberty has been found in essentially all cases old enough to be ascertained for this feature. Hydrocephaly has been found in three cases. Hypotonia and hyperextensible joints have been found in early childhood and may be associated with delayed motor milestones. Overall cognitive function based on formal standardized psychometrics has been in the normal range in a small number of cases so tested. Obesity and Prader–Willi-like phenotype has been described in two cases. Maturity onset diabetes of the young (MODY) was present in a young male with maternal UPD (14). Isodisomy, presence of two copies of one homologue, allowed expression of autosomal recessive rod monochromacy in one case.

PATERNAL UPD (14): Two cases of paternal UPD (14) have been described. Craniofacial malformations were striking and mental retardation was more severe than in maternal UPD (14) cases.

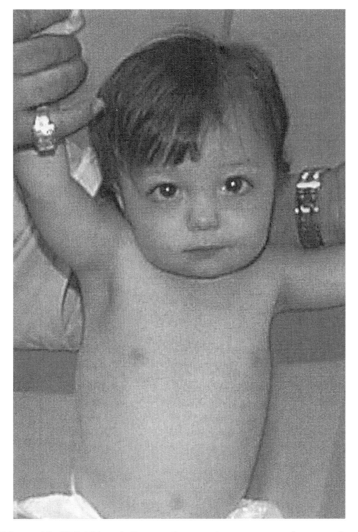

A 12-month-old boy with UPD14(mat). Proportionate short stature, absence of malformation, and normal development are the clinical features of this patient diagnosed at birth due to low birth weight and hypotonia.

CYTOGENETICS: UPD (14) results from the loss of the extra chromosome 14 in a trisomic embryo in some cases, while in others isochromosome 14 and Robertsonian translocations involving the two homologues has been the cause. Segmental or interstitial uniparental disomy of band 14q31 has been reported in one case. Imprinting effects are suspected based on differences noted in the phenotype of maternal versus paternal UPD (14) and evidence of synteny between human chromosome 14 and mouse chromosome 12 on which imprinted loci have been well documented.

REFERENCES

Berends MJ, Hordijk R, Scheffer H, Oosterwijk JC, Halley DJ, Sorgedrager N. 1999. Two cases of maternal uniparental disomy 14 with a phenotype overlapping with the Prader-Willi phenotype. *Am. J. Med. Genet.* 84:76–79.

Eggermann T, Mergenthaler S, Eggermann K, Albers A, Linnemann K, Fusch C, Ranke MB, Wollmann HA. 2001. Identification of interstitial maternal uniparental disomy (UPD) (14) and complete maternal UPD (20) in a cohort of growth retarded patients. *J. Med. Genet.* 38:86–89.

Engel E. 1980. A new genetic concept: uniparental disomy and its potential effect, isodisomy. *Am. J. Med. Genet.* 6: 137–143.

Hordijk R, Wierenga H, Scheffer H, Leegte B, Hofstra RM, Stolte-Dijkstra I. 1999. Maternal uniparental disomy for chromosome 14 in a boy with a normal karyotype. *J. Med. Genet.* 36:782–785.

Manzoni MF, Pramparo T, Stroppolo A, Chiaino F, Bosi E, Zuffardi O, Carrozzo R. 2000. A patient with maternal chromosome 14 UPD presenting with a mild phenotype and MODY. *Clin. Genet.* 57:406–408.

Mignon-Ravix C, Mugneret F, Stavropoulou C, Depetris D, Van Kien PK, Mattei MG. 2001. Maternally inherited duplication of the possible imprinted 14q31 region. *J. Med. Genet.* 38:343–347.

Papenhausen PR, Mueller OT, Johnson VP, Sutcliffe M, Diamond TM, Kousseff BG. 1995. Uniparental isodisomy of chromosome 14 in two cases: an abnormal child and a normal adult. *Am. J. Med. Genet.* 59:271–275.

Pentao L, Lewis RA, Ledbetter DH, Patel PI, Lupski JR. 1992. Maternal uniparental isodisomy of chromosome 14: association with autosomal recessive rod monochromacy. *Am. J. Hum. Genet.* 50:690–699.

Sutton VR, Shaffer LG. 2000. Search for imprinted regions on chromosome 14: comparison of maternal and paternal UPD cases with cases of chromosome 14 deletion. *Am. J. Med. Genet.* 93:381–387.

Tomkins DJ, Roux AF, Waye J, Freeman VC, Cox DW, Whelan D. 1996. Maternal uniparental isodisomy of human chromosome 14 associated with a paternal t(13q14q) and precocious puberty. *Eur. J. Hum. Genet.* 4:153–159.

Wang JC, Passage MB, Yen PH, Shapiro LJ, Mohandas TK. 1991. Uniparental heterodisomy for chromosome 14 in a phenotypically abnormal familial balanced 13/14 Robertsonian translocation carrier. *Am. J. Hum. Genet.* 48:1069–1074.

CHROMOSOME 15 TRISOMY

Trisomy 15 is rarely seen in live births. It is not uncommon in first trimester pregnancy losses and chorionic villi sampled for prenatal diagnosis. The information summarized here is based on six live-born infants and five fetuses: eight females, two males, and one case of unknown sex.

GENERAL CHARACTERISTICS: Growth retardation was noted on three occasions. Developmental delay was noted in all six live-born infants.

ABNORMALITIES

Craniofacies: Prominent forehead, upturned nose, broad nasal bridge (5), cleft soft palate (2), small mouth (4), micrognathia (4), ears described as normal (5), short, thick neck (4)

Limbs: Clenched hands, overlapping fingers, tibial deviation of toes, and clubfoot

Organs: Congenital heart defects were present in four cases. Anteriorly displaced anus, widely spaced nipples, 11 pairs of ribs, fetal hydrops are other anomalies seen.

CYTOGENETICS: All but two cases have been mosaics with a diploid cell line present in varying frequencies in multiple tissues studied. Meiosis I nondisjunction and maternal-age effect have been documented.

PRENATAL DIAGNOSIS OF TRISOMY 15: Trisomy 15 is not uncommon in chorionic villas samples (CVS). In the European collaborative study (EUCROMIC) the incidence was 0.027%. In that study most cases were confined placental mosaicism. Fetal trisomy 15 was found in 1 out of 28 cases in that study. The rest were confined to the cytotrophoblasts, mesodermal stem cells, or found in both types of cells. Amniocentesis is necessary in every case to look for true fetal trisomy 15. Mosaicism may be impossible to exclude with certainty in prenatal cases. Uniparental disomy (UPD) is also possible and should be looked for. Angelman syndrome due to UPD(15)pat and Prader-Willi syndrome due to UPD(15)mat have been described. Intrauterine growth retardation (IUGR) without detectable fetal aneuploidy may also occur secondary to placental insufficiency. Fetal hydrops has been associated with fetal trisomy 15.

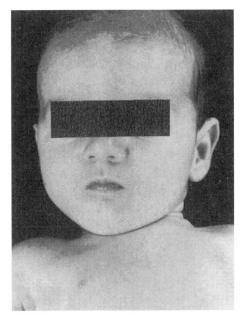

a

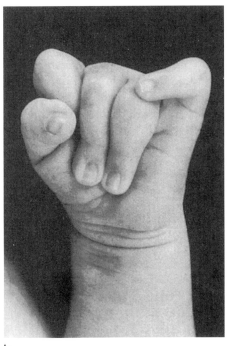

b

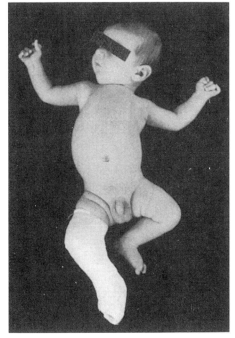

c

Facial features (a), hand posture (b), and foot abnormality (c) of a patient with low-level mosaicism for trisomy 15. (From Buhler et al., 1996. *Am. J. Med. Genet.* 62:109–112. Copyright © 1996 John Wiley & Sons, Inc. Reprinted by permission of Wiley-Liss, Inc.)

REFERENCES

Bennett CP, Davis T, Seller MJ. 1992. Trisomy 15 mosaicism in an IVF fetus. *J. Med. Genet.* 29:745–746.

Buhler EM, Bienz G, Straumann E, Bosch N. 1996. Delineation of a clinical syndrome caused by mosaic trisomy 15. *Am. J. Med. Genet.* 62:109–112.

Eurpoean Collaborative Research on Mosaicism in CVS (EUCROMIC). 1999. Trisomy 15 CPM: probable origins, pregnancy outcome and risk of fetal UPD: European Collaborative Research on Mosaicism in CVS (EUCROMIC). *Prenat. Diagn.* 19:29–35.

Fryns JP, Kleczkowska A, Lagae L, Kenis H, van den Berghe H. 1993. A specific phenotype associated with trisomy 15 mosaicism. *Ann. Genet.* 36:129–131.

Harpey JP, Heron D, Prudent M, Lesourd S, Henry I, Royer-Legrain G, Munnich A, Bonnefont JP. 1998. Recurrent meiotic nondisjunction of maternal chromosome 15 in a sibship. *Am. J. Med. Genet.* 76:103–104.

Kuller JA, Laifer SA. 1991. Trisomy 15 associated with nonimmune hydrops. *Am. J. Perinatol.* 8:39–40.

Markovic VD, Chitayat DA, Ritchie SM, Chodakowski BA, Hutton EM. 1996. Trisomy 15 mosaic derived from trisomic conceptus: report of a case and a review. *Am. J. Med. Genet.* 61:363–370.

Robinson WP, Kuchinka BD, Bernasconi F, Petersen MB, Schulze A, Brondum-Nielsen K, Christian SL, Ledbetter DH, Schinzel AA, Horsthemke B, Schuffenhauer S, Michaelis RC, Langlois S, Hassold TJ. 1998. Maternal meiosis I non-disjunction of chromosome 15: dependence of the maternal age effect on level of recombination. *Hum. Mol. Genet.* 7:1011–1019.

Sundberg K, Brocks V, Jacobsen JR, Beck B. 1994. True trisomy 15 mosaicism, detected by amniocentesis at 12 weeks of gestation and fetal echocardiography. *Prenat. Diagn.* 14:559–563.

CHROMOSOME 15q PROXIMAL TRISOMY

Duplications of the proximal segments of chromosome 15q have been detected in a variety of clinical settings. Cytogenetically visible structural changes involving bands 15q11q12 have been detected in studies of individuals with developmental delay, Prader-Willi syndrome, Angelman syndrome, mental retardation, and autism. Bisatellited supernumerary marker chromosomes found in amniotic fluid samples are frequently derived from chromosome 15 as inverted duplications or isodicentric chromosomes. Such markers are often found to be familial and also detected in phenotypically normal or abnormal relatives of the patient.

With the advent of molecular analysis some of the confusion surrounding the relationship between these chromosomal abnormalities and their phenotypic effects are beginning to be clarified.

The high frequency of chromosome 15 involvement in duplications or even triplications relative to the other acrocentrics is due to the presence of pericentromeric duplicons and other polymorphic variations in the pericentromeric chromatin of chromosome 15. These structural alterations facilitate unequal crossover between the 15 homologues or the two chromatids of a chromosome 15. If the duplications involve the Prader-Willi/Angelman critical region (PWACR), the parent-of-origin effect may determine the phenotype.

Maternally transmitted duplications of 15q11q12 that include the PWACR appear to be related to the autistic spectrum disorders and pervasive developmental delay. Paternally transmitted lesions may not have a specific phenotype. De novo duplications have been found in phenotypically abnormal individuals. No malformations are associated with dup(15)(q11q12).

Clinical interpretation for counseling purposes requires that each dup(15)(q11q12) be evaluated at a minimum for the presence or absence of the PWACR within the duplication and parental studies to determine inheritance pattern, if any.

REFERENCES

Browne CE, Dennis NR, Maher E, Long FL, Nicholson JC, Sillibourne J, Barber JC. 1997. Inherited interstitial duplications of proximal 15q: genotype-phenotype correlations. *Am. J. Hum. Genet.* 61:1342–1352.

Cook EH Jr, Lindgren V, Leventhal BL, Courchesne R, Lincoln A, Shulman C, Lord C, Courchesne E. 1997. Autism or atypical autism in maternally but not paternally derived proximal 15q duplication. *Am. J. Hum. Genet.* 60:928–934.

Kotzot D, Martinez MJ, Bagci G, Basaran S, Baumer A, Binkert F, Brecevic L, Castellan C, Chrzanowska K, Dutly F, Gutkowska A, Karauzum SB, Krajewska-Walasek M, Luleci G, Miny P, Riegel M, Schuffenhauer S, Seidel H, Schinzel A. 2000. Parental origin and mechanisms of formation of cytogenetically recognisable de novo direct and inverted duplications. *J. Med. Genet.* 37:281–286.

Mao R, Jalal SM. 2000. Characteristics of two cases with dup(15)(q11.2–q12): one of maternal and one of paternal origin. *Genet. Med.* 2:131–135.

Repetto GM, White LM, Bader PJ, Johnson D, Knoll JH. 1998. Interstitial duplications of chromosome region 15q11q13: clinical and molecular characterization. *Am. J. Med. Genet.* 79:82–89.

Schroer RJ, Phelan MC, Michaelis RC, Crawford EC, Skinner SA, Cuccaro M, Simensen RJ, Bishop J, Skinner C, Fender D, Stevenson RE. 1998. Autism and maternally derived aberrations of chromosome 15q. *Am. J. Med. Genet.* 76:327–336.

CHROMOSOME 15q PARTIAL MONOSOMY
Non-Prader-Willi 15q Deletion Syndrome

Interstitial deletions of 15q11q12 are most frequently associated with the Prader-Willi syndrome or Angelman syndrome; however, many patients have been reported with 15q deletions involving the same or more distal segments who do not manifest features of either of these syndromes. This summary is based on a review of 25 published cases.

GENERAL CHARACTERISTICS: Mental retardation or developmental delay was present in 92% of the cases.

ABNORMALITIES

Craniofacies: The facial features are not particularly striking. Dysplastic ears (32%), hypertelorism (16%), highly arched palate (28%) are reported in some of the patients. Craniosynostosis was noted on occasion.

Limbs: Small hands with simian creases (25%) and short fingers have been reported.

Other: Hypotonia and other neurological abnormalities (72%) and failure to thrive are described in infancy. Cryptorchidism may be present in 44% of the males. Congenital heart defects (28%), bifid uvula, and skeletal anomalies were less common. Four of 25 patients died during infancy.

CYTOGENETICS: Most cases were secondary to malsegregation of parental translocations involving another autosome. The imbalance resulting from the second chromosome involved in the translocation accounts for some of the variability noted in this syndrome. Precise phenotype–karyotype correlations beyond the absence of Prader-Willi syndrome features have not been defined at this time. The breakpoints and the extent of the monosomy have also varied among the reported cases.

REFERENCES

Autio S, Pihko H, Tengstrom C. 1988. Clinical features in a de novo interstitial deletion 15q13 to q15. *Clin. Genet.* 34:293–298.

Clark RD. 1984. Del(15)(q22q24) syndrome with Potter sequence. *Am. J. Med. Genet.* 19:703–705.

Formiga LD, Poenaru L, Couronne F, Flori E, Eibel JL, Deminatti MM, Savary JB, Lai JL, Gilgenkrantz S, Pierson M. 1988. Interstitial deletion of chromosome 15: two cases. *Hum. Genet.* 80:401–404.

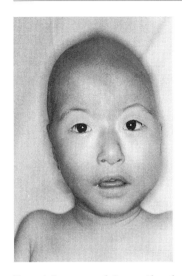 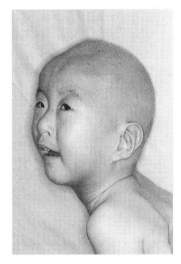 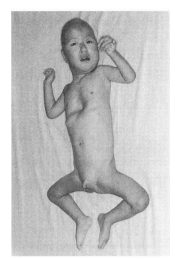

Boy at 1 year and 8 months showing turricephaly, arched eyebrows, shallow orbits, flat nasal bridge, hypoplastic alae nasi, and retrognathia. He was hypotonic and had a developmental quotient of 22. Karyotype was 46,XY,del(15)(q15q22.1). (From Fukushima et al., 1990. *Am. J. Med. Genet.* 36:209–213. Copyright © 1990 John Wiley & Sons, Inc. Reprinted by permission of Wiley-Liss, Inc.)

Fukushima Y, Wakui K, Nishida T, Nishimoto H. 1990. Craniosynostosis in an infant with an interstitial deletion of 15q [46,XY,del(15)(q15q22.1)]. *Am. J. Med. Genet.* 36:209–213.

Galan F, Aguilar MS, Gonzalez J, Clemente F, Sanchez R, Tapia M, Moya M. 1991. Interstitial 15q deletion without a classic Prader-Willi phenotype. *Am. J. Med. Genet.* 38:532–534.

Greenberg F, Ledbetter DH. 1987. Deletions of proximal 15q without Prader-Willi syndrome. *Am. J. Med. Genet.* 28:813–820.

Kaplan LC, Wharton R, Elias E, Mandell F, Donlon T, Latt SA. 1987. Clinical heterogeneity associated with deletions in the long arm of chromosome 15: report of 3 new cases and their possible genetic significance. *Am. J. Med. Genet.* 28:45–53.

Mizuguchi M, Tsukamoto K, Suzuki Y, Nakagome Y. 1994. Myoclonic epilepsy and a maternally derived deletion of 15pter → q13. *Clin. Genet.* 45:44–47.

Pauli RM, Meisner LF, Szmanda RJ. 1983. 'Expanded' Prader-Willi syndrome in a boy with an unusual 15q chromosome deletion. *Am. J. Dis. Child.* 137:1087–1089.

Schwartz S, Max SR, Panny SR, Cohen MM. 1985. Deletions of proximal 15q and non-classical Prader-Willi syndrome phenotypes. *Am. J. Med. Genet.* 20:255–263.

Stewart FJ, Carson DJ, Thomas PS, Humphreys M, Thornton C, Nevin NC. 1996. Wolcott-Rallison syndrome associated with congenital malformations and a mosaic deletion 15q 11–12. *Clin. Genet.* 49:152–155.

ANGELMAN SYNDROME

First described in 1965 by Angelman, the syndrome has an estimated incidence of about 1:15,000 to 1:20,000 live births. The characteristic craniofacial features and neurological and behavioral profile make this a recognizable syndrome in adults as well as children as young as 2 years old. It is caused by lack of maternally imprinted gene functions localized to the proximal 15q11q13 bands in proximity to the Prader-Willi syndrome region.

ABNORMALITIES

Physical: Newborns with Angelman syndrome are normal in appearance and in every other way. Head growth begins to decelerate toward the end of the first year. Older children typically show microcephaly, brachycephaly, flat occiput, large mouth, protruding tongue and the overall appearance of being happy. Final adult stature is below average. Malformations are rare. Strabismus may be present. Hypopigmentation of the eyes is common and includes the iris as well as the fundus. The overall complexion may be lighter than expected for the family background in some patients.

Neurological: Seizure disorders are seen in about 90% of the patients by 3 years of age and associated with abnormal EEG even with good control of clinical seizures. Movement and balance are impaired with gait described as broad-based, unsteady, ataxic, and jerky or puppet-like. Deep tendon reflexes may be hyperactive in the lower limbs.

Behavioral: Inappropriate laughter, paroxysmal bursts of laughter without reason, and a happy predisposition are typical, beginning as early as infancy and persisting into adulthood. Attention deficit and hyperactivity are common. Cognitive deficits are severe and independent adult living is not achieved. Conversational speech never develops. Receptive language and nonverbal communication skills are better preserved.

CYTOGENETICS: Angelman syndrome can result from several mechanisms that lead to the loss of maternally imprinted gene function. Deletions within bands 15q11q13 of the maternally derived chromosomes are detected by fluorescence in situ hybridization (FISH) tests in about 70% of the cases. These have <1% risk of recurrence if the mother's chromosomes are normal.

Paternal uniparental disomy is found in about 5% of the cases. Recurrence risk is <1%. Structural abnormalities of mother's chromosome 15, inherited mutations within the ubiquitin-protein ligase 3A (UBE3A) gene or other mutations that affect the imprinting center (IC) will carry a recurrence risk as high as 50%. De novo mutations carry a low risk.

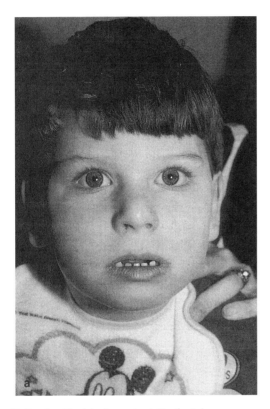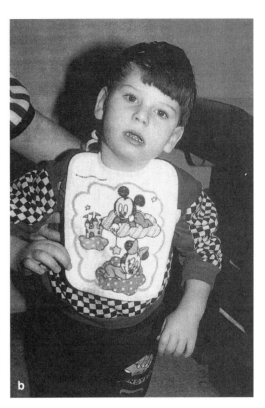

Patient with (a) characteristic facial appearance and (b) gait associated with Angelman syndrome. Microcephaly, seizure and developmental delay were the presenting complaints.

Prenatal diagnosis is possible by combined use of the cytogenetic and molecular methods for families identified to be at risk. These include parents who have had a child with Angelman syndrome, regardless of cause, women identified with trisomy 15 in chorionic villus sampling (CVS) performed for other risks, and those with chromosomal translocations involving chromosome bands 15pter → q13.

REFERENCES

American Society of Human Genetics/American College of Medical Genetics Test and Technology Transfer Committee. 1996. Diagnostic testing for Prader-Willi and Angleman syndromes: Report of the ASHG/ACMG Test and Technology Transfer Committee. *Am. J. Hum. Genet.* 58:1085–1088.

Angelman H. 1965. 'Puppet children': a report of three cases. *Dev. Med. Child Neurol.* 7:681–688.

Buiting K, Barnicoat A, Lich C, Pembrey M, Malcolm S, Horsthemke B. 2001. Disruption of the bipartite imprinting center in a family with Angelman syndrome. *Am. J. Hum. Genet.* 68:1290–1294.

Buntinx IM, Hennekam RC, Brouwer OF, Stroink H, Beuten J, Mangelschots K, Fryns JP. 1995. Clinical profile of Angelman syndrome at different ages. *Am. J. Med. Genet.* 56:176–183.

Burger J, Buiting K, Dittrich B, Gross S, Lich C, Sperling K, Horsthemke B, Reis A. 1997. Different mechanisms and recurrence risks of imprinting defects in Angelman syndrome. *Am. J. Hum. Genet.* 61:88–93.

Moncla A, Malzac P, Voelckel MA, Auquier P, Girardot L, Mattei MG, Philip N, Mattei JF, Lalande M, Livet MO. 1999. Phenotype-genotype correlation in 20 deletion and 20 non-deletion Angelman syndrome patients. *Eur. J. Hum. Genet.* 7:131–139.

Ohta T, Buiting K, Kokkonen H, McCandless S, Heeger S, Leisti H, Driscoll DJ, Cassidy SB, Horsthemke B, Nicholls RD. 1999. Molecular mechanism of angelman syndrome in two large families involves an imprinting mutation. *Am. J. Hum. Genet.* 64:385–396.

Sandanam T, Beange H, Robson L, Woolnough H, Buchholz T, Smith A. 1997. Manifestations in institutionalised adults with Angelman syndrome due to deletion. *Am. J. Med. Genet.* 70:415–420.

Stalker HJ, Williams CA. 1998. Genetic counseling in Angelman syndrome: the challenges of multiple causes. *Am. J. Med. Genet.* 77:54–59.

Williams CA, Lossie A, Driscoll D; R.C. Phillips Unit. 2001. Angelman syndrome: mimicking conditions and phenotypes. *Am. J. Med. Genet.* 101:59–64.

PRADER-WILLI SYNDROME

First described in 1956, Prader-Willi syndrome (PWS) has an estimated incidence of about 1 in 10,000 to 1 in 15,000 births. Its primary manifestations include hypothalamic dysfunction, minor dysmorphism, and a characteristic behavioral profile. The disorder results from lack of paternally imprinted gene functions localized to the Prader-Willi/Angelman critical region on 15q11q12. In addition to being relatively common, PWS is important as a model for an increasing number of disorders in which imprinting and other complex epigenetic phenomena will necessitate greater levels of sophistication from clinicians involved in their diagnosis and treatment.

MAIN FEATURES: Neonatal hypotonia, failure to thrive, childhood obesity, short stature

GENERAL CHARACTERISTICS: The syndrome can be diagnosed in newborns and young infants on the basis of generalized hypotonia and its consequences such as poor suck and failure to thrive, especially if associated with the dysmorphic features described below.

ABNORMALITIES

Craniofacies: Reduced bitemporal diameter, almond-shaped eyes, small mouth, trapezoid-shaped mouth with downturned corners.

Limbs: Small hands with puffy dorsum, tapering fingers, straight ulnar border of hands.

Genitourinary: Genital hypoplasia manifested as cryptorchidism, hypoplastic scrotum, small penis in the male and clitoral hypoplasia in the female are recognizable in newborns and persist through adulthood. Puberty is delayed and inadequate. Hypogonadism is of hypothalamic/pituitary origin and responds to hormone therapy. Infertility is virtually constant with only exceptional cases of reproduction reported in females.

Performance: The best-known and consistent behavioral abnormality is food seeking, foraging for food, pica, and lack of satiety, which may contribute to obesity. Temper tantrums, stubbornness, and skin picking are also common behavioral traits. Pain threshold may be high. Overall cognitive ability is reduced. Measured IQ scores tend to be in borderline normal to mildly retarded range. Psychotic disorders are more prevalent in adolescents and adults with PWS.

Other: In older children and adults, truncal obesity associated with short stature, small hands and feet, straight ulnar border of the hands, hypotonia, scoliosis, and kyphosis are common. Growth hormone deficiency and good response to growth hormone therapy have been documented. Hypopigmentation of the eyes and skin

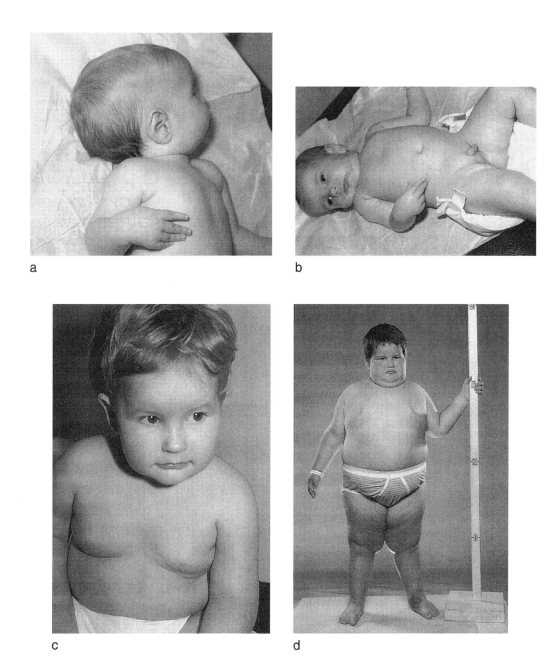

Patient 1 showing the evolution of the Prader-Willi syndrome from birth to age 4 years. Notice (a) micrognathia, occipital prominence, puffy hands with tapering fingers (b) undescended testes and underdeveloped penis (c) excessive weight gain beginning in the second year and (d) morbid obesity by age 4 years.

relative to family background is reported in about 30% of the patients. Thick, ropy saliva is considered a unique feature of PWS and may be a contributing factor in excessive dental caries and speech articulation problems.

CYTOGENETICS: Consensus diagnostic criteria and an objective scoring system are available to identify cases that require laboratory testing. The laboratory testing of PWS is somewhat complex because PWS can result from several mechanisms. Large interstitial deletions within the Prader-Willi/Angelman critical region (PWACR) account for about 70% of the cases. Fluorescence in situ hybridization (FISH) test will identify those cases. High-resolution karyotyping may reveal some of these deletions but cannot be relied on for diagnostic purposes.

A methylation-based assay is used to demonstrate "maternal inheritance only" pattern indicating deletion within paternal 15 or uniparental disomy (UPD[15]) mat when additional probes and comparison with both parents are possible. Small deletions or other structural changes that cause imprinting center dysfunction are identified by inclusion of additional probes for FISH testing and karyotype results. A small number, <1% of the cases, may still remain unrecognized. Genetic recurrence risk varies. For parents of children with PWS due to a large deletion or UPD the recurrence risk is low (1% or less). For those with imprinting center dysfunction the recurrence risk may be high. Prenatal testing for PWS is possible.

Several excellent reviews of the clinical phenotype, diagnosis, etiology and management, as well as position papers on recommended diagnostic strategies are listed in the References.

REFERENCES

Butler MG. 1989. Hypopigmentation: a common feature of Prader-Labhart-Willi syndrome. *Am. J. Hum. Genet.* 45:140–146.

Carrel AL, Myers SE, Whitman BY, Allen DB. 1999. Growth hormone improves body composition, fat utilization, physical strength and agility, and growth in Prader-Willi syndrome: a controlled study. *J. Pediatr.* 134:215–221.

Cassidy SB. 1997. Prader-Willi syndrome. *J. Med. Genet.* 34:917–923.

Cassidy SB, Beaduet AL, Knoll JHM, Ledbetter DH, Nichols RD, Schwartz S, Butler MG, Watson M. 1996. Diagnostic testing for Prader-Willi and Angleman syndromes: report of the ASHG/ACMG Test and Technology Transfer Committee. *Am. J. Hum. Genet.* 58:1085–1088.

Gillessen-Kaesbach G, Robinson W, Lohmann D, Kaya-Westerloh S, Passarge E, Horsthemke B. 1995. Genotype-phenotype correlation in a series of 167 deletion and non-deletion patients with Prader-Willi syndrome. *Hum. Genet.* 96:638–643.

Holm VA, Cassidy SB, Butler MG, Hanchett JM, Greenswag LR, Whitman BY, Greenberg F. 1993. Prader-Willi syndrome: consensus diagnostic criteria. *Pediatrics* 91:398–402.

Kuslich CD, Kobori JA, Mohapatra G, Gregorio-King C, Donlon TA. 1999. Prader-Willi syndrome is caused by disruption of the SNRPN gene. *Am. J. Hum. Genet.* 64:70–76.

Ledbetter DH, Riccardi VM, Airhart SD, Strobel RJ, Keenan BS, Crawford JD. 1981. Deletions of chromosome 15 as a cause of the Prader-Willi syndrome. *N. Engl. J. Med.* 304:325–329.

Lindgren AC, Hellstrom LG, Ritzen EM, Milerad J. 1999. Growth hormone treatment increases CO(2) response, ventilation and central inspiratory drive in children with Prader-Willi syndrome. *Eur. J. Pediatr.* 158:936–940.

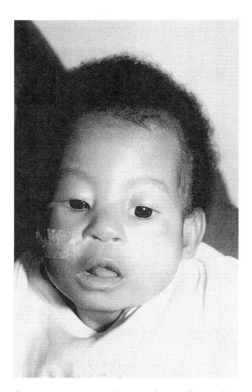

African-American female infant at age 4 months. Prader-Willi syndrome diagnosed at birth because of intrauterine growth retardation, marked neonatal hypotonia and almond-shaped eyes. Notice naso-gastric feeding tube required for maintenance of adequate intake.

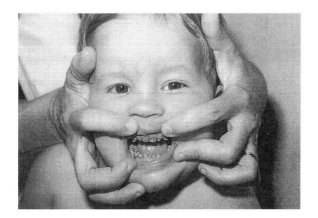

Patient 1 showing discolored and carious teeth.

RING CHROMOSOME 15

A clinical syndrome due to ring 15 has been described on the basis of more than 35 observations.

MAIN FEATURES: Prenatal and postnatal growth retardation, mental retardation

GENERAL CHARACTERISTICS: Mental retardation is nearly always present but variable in severity. Reduced birth length (<46 cm.) was noted in 70% of the cases. Short stature was present in 90% of the children and adults.

ABNORMALITIES

Craniofacies: Microcephaly is the most common finding present in 80% of the patients. Brachycephaly, hypertelorism, hypotelorism, triangular facies, broad nasal bridge, anomalous pinnae, micrognathia, and highly arched palate occur in at least a third of all cases.

Limbs: Small hands, transverse palmar crease, fifth-finger clinodactyly, talipes equinovarus, and syndactyly of the second and third toes have been noted in 10% to 25% of the cases.

Other: Congenital heart defects and renal malformations have been found in 20% and 5% of the cases, respectively. Similarity to the Russell–Silver syndrome has been noted more than once. Good response to growth hormone therapy has been documented. Mental retardation is constant but variable in severity with "nearly normal intelligence" found in some patients. Café-au-lait spots, hypopigmented spots are an occasional finding. Rarely cryptorchidism and hypospadias have been noted in males. Azoospermia and infertility have been reported in several adult males. Females are fertile and have transmitted the ring chromosome to offspring.

CLINICAL COURSE: Life expectancy for r(15) patients is unknown, but may be normal in the absence of major congenital heart defects. Many adult patients have been reported.

CYTOGENETICS: Mosaicism and extent of the monosomy secondary to the breakpoints involved in ring formation influence the phenotypic expression. Most cases are sporadic, but familial occurrence has been documented.

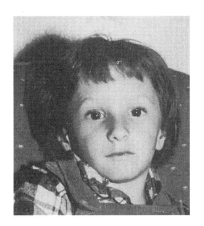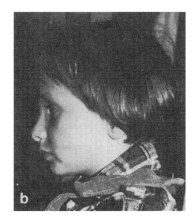

Boy 3 years and 7 months of age with r(15). Note triangular face and micrognathia. (From Butler et al., 1988. *Am. J. Med. Genet.* 29:140–154. Copyright © 1988 John Wiley & Sons, Inc. Reprinted by permission of Wiley-Liss, Inc.)

REFERENCES

Butler MG, Fogo AB, Fuchs DA, Collins FS, Dev VG, Phillips JA 3rd. 1988. Two patients with ring chromosome 15 syndrome. *Am. J. Med. Genet.* 29:149–154.

de Jong G, Rossouw RA, Retief AE. 1989. Ring chromosome 15 in a patient with features of Fryns' syndrome. *J. Med. Genet.* 26:469–470.

Fryns JP, Kleczkowska A, Buttiens M, Jonckheere P, Brouckmans-Buttiens K, van den Berghe H. 1986. Ring chromosome 15 syndrome: further delineation of the adult phenotype. *Ann. Genet.* 29:45–48.

Horigome Y, Kondo I, Kuwajima K, Suzuki T. 1992. Familial occurrence of ring chromosome 15. *Clin. Genet.* 41:178–180.

Kousseff BG. 1980. Ring chromosome 15 and failure to thrive. *Am. J. Dis. Child.* 134:798–799.

Kitatani M, Takahashi H, Ozaki M, Okino E, Maruoka T. 1990. A case of ring chromosome 15 accompanied by almost normal intelligence. *Hum. Genet.* 85:138–139.

Laszlo J, Gaal M, Bosze P. 1982. Primary gonadal hypoplasia and dysmorphic features in ring chromosome 15 syndrome. *Clin. Genet.* 21:351.

Matsuishi T, Yamada Y, Endo K, Sakai H, Fukushima Y. 1996. Ring chromosome 15 syndrome in an adult female. *J. Intellect. Disabil. Res.* 40:478–480.

Meinecke P, Koske-Westphal T. 1980. Ring chromosome 15 in a male adult with radial defects: evaluation of the phenotype. *Clin. Genet.* 18:428–433.

Moreau N, Teyssier M. 1982. Ring chromosome 15: report of a case in an infertile man. *Clin. Genet.* 21:272–279.

Nuutinen M, Kouvalainen K, Knip M. 1995. Good growth response to growth hormone treatment in the ring chromosome 15 syndrome. *J. Med. Genet.* 32:486–487.

Otto J, Back E, Furste HO, Abel M, Bohm N, Pringsheim W. 1984. Dysplastic features, growth retardation, malrotation of the gut, and fatal ventricular septal defect in a 4-month-old girl with ring chromosome 15. *Eur. J. Pediatr.* 142:229–231.

Rogan PK, Seip JR, Driscoll DJ, Papenhausen PR, Johnson VP, Raskin S, Woodward AL, Butler MG. 1996. Distinct 15q genotypes in Russell-Silver and ring 15 syndromes. *Am. J. Med. Genet.* 62:10–15.

Smith A, den Dulk G, Viersbach R, Michas J. 1991. Ring chromosome 15 and 15qs+ mosaic: clinical and cytogenetic behaviour spanning 29 years. *Am. J. Med. Genet.* 40:460–463.

Wilson GN, Sauder SE, Bush M, Beitins IZ. 1985. Phenotypic delineation of ring chromosome 15 and Russell-Silver syndromes. *J. Med. Genet.* 22:233–236.

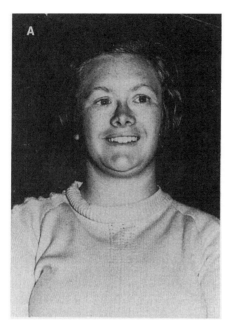
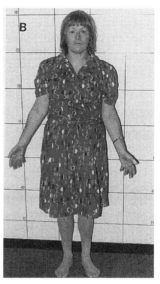
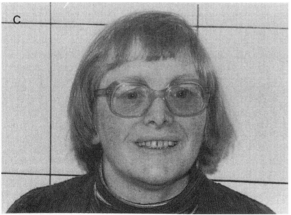
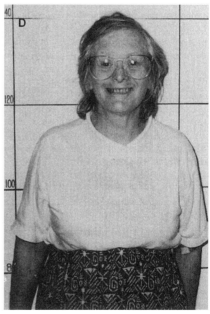

Patient with r(15) at age 26 (A), 30 (B), 48 (C), and 59 (D) years. Note the near-normal phenotype. (From Smith et al., 1991. *Am. J. Med. Genet.* 40:460–463. Copyright © 1991 John Wiley & Sons, Inc. Reprinted by permission of Wiley-Liss, Inc.)

CHROMOSOME 16p PARTIAL TRISOMY

Chromosome 16p trisomy has been described in at least 26 cases. A multiple congenital anomalies/mental retardation syndrome with remarkably similar craniofacial and limb anomalies is apparent.

MAIN FEATURES: Round head, small palpebral fissures, sparse eyebrows and eyelashes

GENERAL CHARACTERISTICS: Most patients are born at term but below average in weight. No pregnancy complications have been particularly common.

ABNORMALITIES

Craniofacies: Anomalies found in >90% of the patients include round head shape, narrow palpebral fissures, sparse eyebrows and eyelashes, hypertelorism, broad nasal bridge, prominent nasal tip, anteverted nares, long philtrum, midline cleft palate, micrognathia, low-set rounded ears with prominent antihelix

Limbs: Overlapping fingers, tapering fingers, simian creases, and clubfoot have been found in 30% to 90% of the patients.

Other: About 50% of the patients had congenital heart defects, respiratory distress, seizures, hypotonia or hypertonia.

CLINICAL COURSE: Mortality was 50% during infancy. Three children reported to be alive at 7, 11, and 15 years old were severely mentally retarded.

CYTOGENETICS: Most cases have been due to unbalanced translocations with the involvement of a number of different autosomes. One case of X/autosome translocation, one with direct tandem duplication, and another with insertion of a 16p segment into 16q have provided opportunities to observe the "pure trisomy 16p" phenotype. These cases did not differ from the others described above in aggregate.

REFERENCES

Carrasco Juan JL, Cigudosa JC, Otero Gomez A, Acosta Almeida MT, Garcia Miranda JL. 1997. De novo trisomy 16p. *Am. J. Med. Genet.* 68:219–221.

Cohen MM, Lerner C, Balkin NE. 1983. Duplication of 16p from insertion of 16p into 16q with subsequent duplication due to crossing over within the inserted segment. *Am. J. Med. Genet.* 14:89–96.

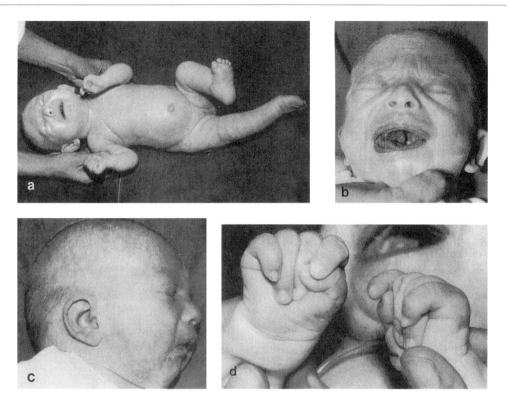

Newborn with 16p trisomy secondary to 46,X,der(X),t(X;16)(q28;p12)mat. (From Preis et al., 1996. *Am. J. Med. Genet.* 61:117–121. Copyright © 1996 John Wiley & Sons, Inc. Reprinted by permission from Wiley-Liss, Inc.)

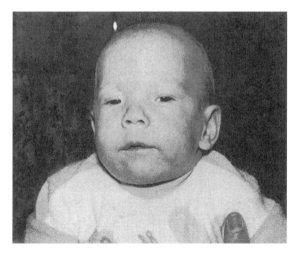

A 6-month-old male with dup(16)(p11.2p12). Note typical facial appearance. (From Carrasco Juan et al., 1997. *Am. J. Med. Genet.* 68:219–221. Copyright © 1997 John Wiley & Sons, Inc. Reprinted by permission from Wiley-Liss, Inc.)

Hebebrand J, Martin M, Korner J, Roitzheim B, de Braganca K, Werner W, Remschmidt H. 1994. Partial trisomy 16p in an adolescent with autistic disorder and Tourette's syndrome. *Am. J. Med. Genet.* 54:268–270.

Houlston RS, Renshaw RM, James RS, Ironton R, Temple IK. 1994. Duplication of 16q22 → qter confirmed by fluorescence in situ hybridisation and molecular analysis. *J. Med Genet.* 31:884–887.

Leonard C, Huret JL, Imbert MC, Lebouc Y, Selva J, Boulley AM. 1992. Trisomy 16p in a liveborn offspring due to maternal translocation t(16;21)(q11;p11) and review of the literature. *Am. J. Med. Genet.* 43:621–625.

Leschot NJ, De Nef JJ, Geraedts JP, Becker-Bloemkolk MJ, Talma A, Bijlsma JB, Verjaal M. 1979. Five familial cases with a trisomy 16p syndrome due to translocation. *Clin. Genet.* 16:205–214.

Mascarello JT, Hubbard V. 1991. Routine use of methods for improved G-band resolution in a population of patients with malformations and developmental delay. *Am. J. Med. Genet.* 38:37–42.

Preis W, Barbi G, Liptay S, Kennerknecht I, Schwemmle S, Pohlandt F. 1996. X/autosome translocation in three generations ascertained through an infant with trisomy 16p due to failure of spreading of X-inactivation. *Am. J. Med. Genet.* 61:117–121.

Roberts SH, Duckett DP. 1978. Trisomy 16p in a liveborn infant and a review of partial and full trisomy 16. *J. Med. Genet.* 15:375–381.

CHROMOSOME 16q PARTIAL TRISOMY

Partial trisomy for the long arm of chromosome 16 has been reported in at least 25 cases: 14 males, 10 females, and one of unknown sex. Most were secondary to malsegregation of balanced translocations involving several different autosomes.

MAIN FEATURES: Severe mental retardation, poor growth, prominent forehead, small palpebral fissures.

GENERAL CHARACTERISTICS: Low birth weight and postnatal failure to thrive have been present in virtually all survivors.

ABNORMALITIES

Craniofacies: A prominent, high forehead, abnormal skull shape, small palpebral fissures, and low-set, dysplastic ears were noted in >80% of the cases. Broad, deformed nasal bridge, antimongoloid slant, and thin upper lip were present in 50–75% of the cases. Micrognathia was also common (about 60%).

Limbs: Flexion contractures of fingers and other joints, fifth-finger clinodactyly, clubfoot, and joint dislocation were found in 50–60% of the cases.

Organs: Congenital heart defects (50%), cryptorchidism, genital hypoplasia, ambiguous genitalia, gastrointestinal anomalies, and choanal stenosis in descending order of frequency

CLINICAL COURSE: More than 50% died in infancy. At least one adult has been reported. This 28-year-old male had short stature, severe mental retardation, and behavioral problems, including self-mutilation.

CYTOGENETICS: All but four cases were due to translocations. Maternal as well as paternal transmission has occurred. Those trisomic for the entire long arm and those trisomic for only the distal 16q21qter bands share similar phenotypic characteristics except greater frequency of internal organ malformations in those trisomic for the larger segment. Four cases of dir dup(16)(q11.2q13) show a different phenotype. They have normal or minimally dysmorphic craniofacial anomalies and no internal organ malformations. However, severe to profound mental retardation was present.

Prenatal diagnosis of a fetus karyotyped because of anomalies detected by ultrasound has been reported.

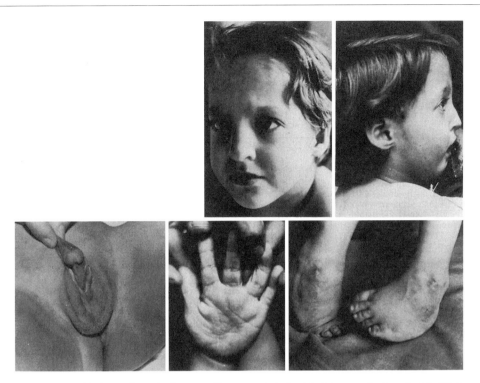

Facial appearance, limb, and genital anomalies associated with trisomy for bands 16q22qter and monosomy for 11p15pter. (From Calva et al., 1984. *Ann. Genet.* 27:122–125. Reprinted with permission from Expansion Scientifique Francaise.)

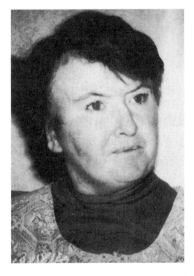

A 34-year-old woman with profound mental retardation, aggressive behavior, and no major anomalies. Her karyotyped was 46, XX, dir dup(16)(q11.2q13) . (From Romain et al., 1984. *Am. J. Med. Genet.* 19:507–513. Copyright © 1984 John Wiley & Sons, Inc. Reprinted by permission of Wiley-Liss, Inc.)

REFERENCES

Balestrazzi P, Giovannelli G, Landucci Rubini L, Dallapiccola B. 1979. Partial trisomy 16q resulting from maternal translocation. *Hum. Genet.* 49:229–235.

Dallapiccola B, Curatolo P, Balestrazzi P. 1979. 'De novo' trisomy 16q11 to pter. *Hum. Genet.* 49:1–6.

Eggermann T, Kolin-Gerresheim I, Gerresheim F, Schwanitz G. 1998. A case of de novo translocation 16;21: trisomy 16q phenotype and origin of the aberration. *Ann. Genet.* 41:205–208.

Engelen JJ, De Die-Smulders CE, Vos PT, Meers LE, Albrechts JC, Hamers AJ. 1999. Characterization of a partial trisomy 16q with FISH: report of a patient and review of the literature. *Ann. Genet.* 42:101–104.

Fryns JP, Kleczkowska A, Decock P, Van den Berghe H. 1990. Direct duplication 16q11.1 → 16q13 is not associated with a typical dysmorphic syndrome. *Ann. Genet.* 33:46–48.

Houlston RS, Renshaw RM, James RS, Ironton R, Temple IK. 1994. Duplication of 16q22 → qter confirmed by fluorescence in situ hybridisation and molecular analysis. *J. Med. Genet.* 31:884–887.

Paladini D, D'Agostino A, Liguori M, Teodoro A, Tartaglione A, Colombari S, Martinelli P. 1999. Prenatal findings in trisomy 16q of paternal origin. *Prenat. Diagn.* 19:472–475.

Romain DR, Frazer AG, Columbano-Green LM, Parfitt RG, Smythe RH, Chapman CJ. 1984. Direct intrachromosomal duplication of 16q and heritable fragile site fra (10)(q25) in the same patient. *Am. J. Med. Genet.* 19:507–513.

CHROMOSOME 16q PARTIAL MONOSOMY

Partial monosomy for the long arm of chromosome 16 is associated with a syndrome of craniofacial, limb, and musculoskeletal defects and internal malformation involving the heart and kidneys. Mental retardation is present in all cases.

MAIN FEATURES: Prominent nose, dysplastic ears, iris coloboma, cleft palate

GENERAL CHARACTERISTICS: Prenatal and postnatal growth retardation was present in 50% and 80% of the cases, respectively. Failure to thrive and generalized hypotonia were reported in nearly all cases reviewed by Monoghan et al. (1997).

ABNORMALITIES

Craniofacies: Large anterior fontanelle, prominent metopic sutures, high forehead, low-set, dysplastic ears, broad, flat nasal bridge, high-arched or cleft palate or micrognathia were present in 65% to 100% of the cases. Short palpebral fissures, and upward-slanting palpebral fissures were somewhat less frequently noted.

Limbs: Broad great toes, malpositioned toes, flawed fingers, bilateral simian creases, and talipes varus or valgus deformities of the feet were described in descending order of frequency.

Other: Short neck and narrow thorax were common. Congenital heart defects and renal cystic dysplasia were reported in about 40% of the patients.

CLINICAL COURSE: Most reported cases have been infants and children. The oldest patient was 25 years old. There may be a female preponderance. All patients have been severely mentally retarded.

CYTOGENETICS: Most cases are due to interstitial deletions involving various segments. Deletions within the most distal bands 16q23q24 are rarely reported. Deletions involving bands 16q11 and 16q22.2 have been the most frequent. Phenotype and karyotype correlation have been attempted by a number of authors. Unique syndromes attributable to proximal and distal deletions have not yet emerged.

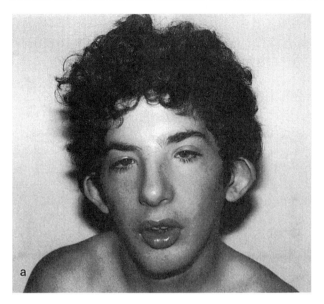
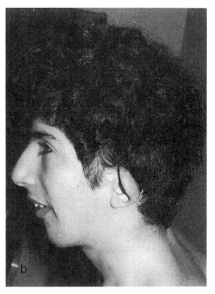

Male with del(16)(q13q22). Note high forehead, short, downward-slanting palpebral fissures, ptosis, cupped, apparently low-set ears, and beaked nose with prominent bridge. (From Casamassima et al., 1990. *Am. J. Med. Genet.* 37:504–509. Copyright © 1990 John Wiley & Sons, Inc. Reprinted by permission from Wiley-Liss, Inc.)

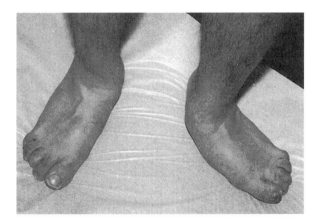

Note the broad great toes and valgus deformity of the left foot. (From Casamassima et al., 1990. *Am. J. Med. Genet.* 37:504–509. Copyright © 1990 John Wiley & Sons, Inc. Reprinted by permission from Wiley-Liss, Inc.)

REFERENCES

Callen DF, Eyre H, Lane S, Shen Y, Hansmann I, Spinner N, Zackai E, McDonald-McGinn D, Schuffenhauer S, Wauters J, et al. 1993. High resolution mapping of interstitial long arm deletions of chromosome 16: relationship to phenotype. *J. Med. Genet.* 30:828–832.

Casamassima AC, Klein RM, Wilmot PL, Brenholz P, Shapiro LR. 1990. Deletion of 16q with prolonged survival and unusual radiographic manifestations. *Am. J. Med. Genet.* 37:504–509.

Chen CP, Chern SR, Lee CC, Chen LF, Chuang CY. 1998. Prenatal diagnosis of de novo interstitial 16q deletion in a fetus associated with sonographic findings of prominent coronal sutures, a prominent frontal bone, and shortening of the long bones. *Prenat. Diagn.* 18:490–495.

Elder FF, Ferguson JW, Lockhart LH. 1984. Identical twins with deletion 16q syndrome: evidence that 16q12.2–q13 is the critical band region. *Hum. Genet.* 67:233–236.

Fujiwara M, Yoshimoto T, Morita Y, Kamada M. 1992. Interstitial deletion of chromosome 16q: 16q22 is critical for 16q-syndrome. *Am. J. Med. Genet.* 43:561–564.

Hoo JJ, Lowry RB, Lin CC, Haslam RH. 1985. Recurrent de novo interstitial deletion of 16q in two mentally retarded sisters. *Clin. Genet.* 27:420–425.

Krauss CM, Caldwell D, Atkins L. 1987. Interstitial deletion and ring chromosome derived from 16q. *J. Med. Genet.* 24:308–312.

Monaghan KG, Van Dyke DL, Wiktor A, Feldman GL. 1997. Cytogenetic and clinical findings in a patient with a deletion of 16q23.1: first report of bilateral cataracts and a 16q deletion. *Am. J. Med. Genet.* 73:180–183.

Naritomi K, Shiroma N, Izumikawa Y, Sameshima K, Ohdo S, Hirayama K. 1988. 16q21 is critical for 16q deletion syndrome. *Clin. Genet.* 33:372–375.

Schuffenhauer S, Callen DF, Seidel H, Shen Y, Lederer G, Murken J. 1992. De novo interstitial deletion 16(q12.1q13) of paternal origin in a 10-year-old boy. *Clin. Genet.* 42:246–250.

Werner W, Kraft S, Callen DF, Bartsch O, Hinkel GK. 1997. A small deletion of 16q23.1 → 16q24.2 [del(16)(q23.1q24.2).ish del(16)(q23.1q24.2)(D16S395+, D16S348−, P5432+)] in a boy with iris coloboma and minor anomalies. *Am. J. Med. Genet.* 70:371–376.

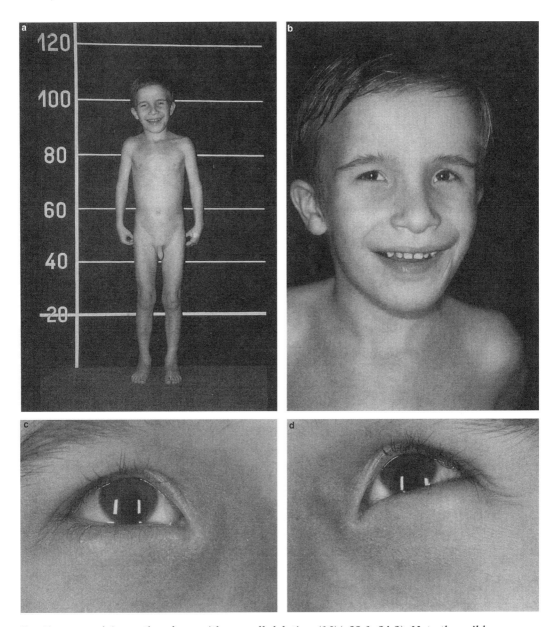

Boy 5 years and 6 months of age with a small deletion (16)(q23.1q24.2). Note the milder phenotype compared to the previous patient with more proximal and larger deletions. (From Werner et al., 1997. *Am. J. Med. Genet.* 70:371–376. Copyright © 1997 John Wiley & Sons, Inc. Reprinted by permission from Wiley-Liss, Inc.)

CHROMOSOME 17p PARTIAL TRISOMY

Trisomy for most or all of the short arm of chromosome 17 has been associated with a distinctive congenital anomalies syndrome. This summary is based on a review of 10 reported cases.

MAIN FEATURES: Mental retardation, microcephaly, malformed pinnae, micrognathia

GENERAL CHARACTERISTICS: Poor prenatal and postnatal growth, developmental delay, and moderate to severe mental retardation are present in all cases except those involving duplication of bands 17p11.2p12 only.

ABNORMALITIES

Craniofacies: Microcephaly (80%), malformed, low-set ears (90%), prominent antihelix, micrognathia (80%), broad nasal bridge (56%), narrow palpebral fissures (40%), and hypertelorism (40%) are the most commonly reported features. Microphthalmia, small pupils have been rarely noted. Highly arched palate was present in 7 of 10 cases.

Limbs: Flexion deformity of fingers, adducted thumbs, long, tapered fingers, simian crease, and distal palmar axial triradius are present in 25% to 70% of the patients.

Other: Short neck with redundant skin, widely spaced nipples, congenital puffy feet reminiscent of Turner syndrome was reason for ascertainment in one case. Hydrocephalus, renal anomalies, inguinal hernia, hiatal hernia, and cryptorchidism were observed in 20% or fewer cases.

CYTOGENETICS: Most cases have been do novo duplications involving most of 17p. Interstitial duplication of bands 17pll.2p12 has been associated with a milder phenotype. At least two patients with 17p duplication showed neuropathological features of Charcot-Marie-Tooth type hereditary sensory motor neuropathy.

REFERENCES

Docherty Z, Hulten MA, Honeyman MM. 1983. De novo tandem duplication 17p11 leads to cen. *J. Med. Genet.* 20:138–142.

Feldman GM, Baumer JG, Sparkes RS. 1982. Brief clinical report: the dup(17p) syndrome. *Am. J. Med. Genet.* 11:299–304.

Kozma C, Meck JM, Loomis KJ, Galindo HC. 1991. De novo duplication of 17p[dup(17)(p12 → p11.2)]: Report of an additional case with confirmation of the cytogenetic, phenotypic, and developmental aspects. *Am. J. Med. Genet.* 41:446–450.

Magenis RE, Brown MG, Allen L, Reiss. 1986. De novo partial duplication of 17p [dup(17)(p12 → p11.2)]: clinical report. *Am. J. Med. Genet.* 24:415–420.

Mascarello JT, Jones MC, Hoyme HE, Freebury MM. 1983. Duplication (17p) in a child with an isodicentric (17p) chromosome. *Am. J. Med. Genet.* 14:67–72.

Roa BB, Greenberg F, Gunaratne P, Sauer CM, Lubinsky MS, Kozma C, Meck JM, Magenis RE, Shaffer LG, Lupski JR. 1996. Duplication of the PMP22 gene in 17p partial trisomy patients with Charcot-Marie-Tooth type-1 neuropathy. *Hum. Genet.* 97:642–649.

Schrander-Stumpel C, Schrander J, Fryns JP, Hamers G. 1990. Trisomy 17p due to a t(8;17)(p23;p11.2)pat translocation: case report and review of the literature. *Clin. Genet.* 37:148–152.

Spinner NB, Biegel JA, Sovinsky L, McDonald-McGinn D, Rehberg K, Parmiter AH, Zackai EH. 1993. 46,XX,15p+ documented as dup(17p) by fluorescence in situ hybridization. *Am. J. Med. Genet.* 46:95–97.

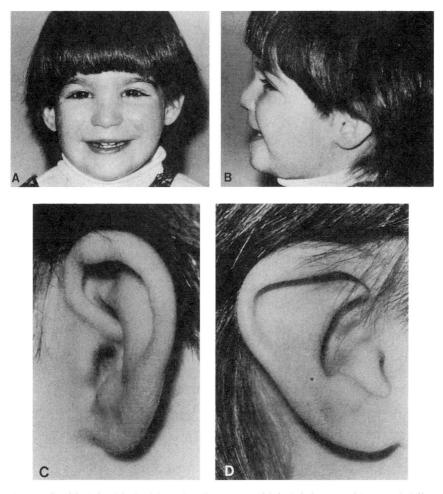

A 2-year 8-month-old girl with (17)(p11.2p12). Note mild facial dysmorphism and different appearance of the two ears. (From Magenis et al., 1986. *Am. J. Med. Genet.* 24:415–420. Copyright © 1986 John Wiley & Sons, Inc. Reprinted by permission of Wiley-Liss, Inc.)

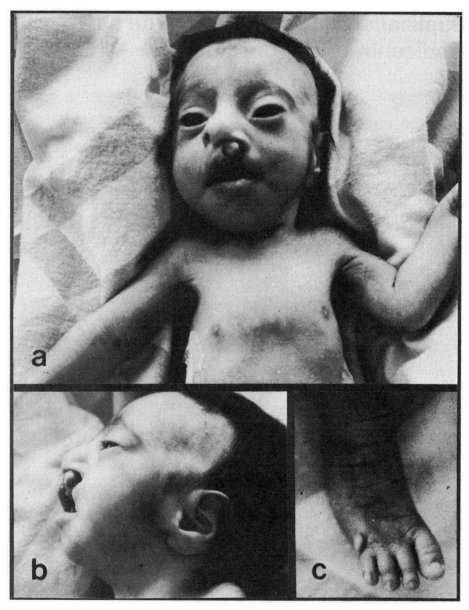

A 4-week-old infant with trisomy for the entire short arm of 17 due to isodicentric 17p. The 17q arm was translocated to 10p15. (From Mascarello et al., 1983. *Am. J. Med. Genet.* 14:67–72. Copyright © 1983 John Wiley & Sons, Inc. Reprinted by permission of Wiley-Liss, Inc.)

CHROMOSOME 17p11.2 MONOSOMY
Smith–Magenis Syndrome

Monosomy for bands 17p11.2 is associated with a recognizable syndrome with somatic, cognitive, and behavioral features known as the Smith–Magenis syndrome (SMS).

MAIN FEATURES: Mild short stature, brachycephaly, flat midface mental retardation, behavioral problems

GENERAL CHARACTERISTICS: Short stature and certain behavioral characteristics are consistent findings and helpful in clinical diagnosis. In addition to self-injurious behaviors common to individuals with mental retardation in general, patients with (SMS) show trichotillomania, sleep disturbances, "self-hugging," and insertion of foreign objects into body orifices with high frequency. Attention-deficit, hyperactivity disorder, destructive and aggressive behavior, explosive outbursts, and temper tantrums are also common. However, children with SMS manifest a calm, cooperative, friendly demeanor most of the time. Mental retardation is always present and can vary in severity from borderline to mild to profound deficits.

ABNORMALITIES

Craniofacies: These abnormalities are usually subtle and consist of brachycephaly, flat midface, depressed nasal bridge, epicanthal folds, and prognathism. Synophrys and ear anomalies may be present.

Limbs: Short, wide hands with brachydactyly, clinodactyly, abnormal palmar creases, and persistent fetal pads on fingertips are seen in 40% to 90% of the cases.

CYTOGENETICS: High-resolution chromosome analysis and fluorescence in situ hybridization (FISH) testing will identify most cases. Almost all reported cases have been sporadic due to de novo deletions within band 17p11.2. An unusual case of intrachromosomal insertion of 17q into 17p11.2 has been reported. Familial SMS due to inheritance from a mother mosaic for 17p11.2 deletion has been reported.

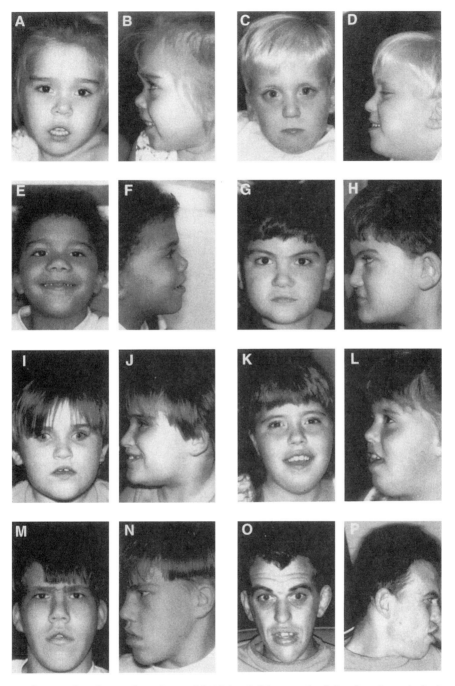

Spectrum of craniofacial manifestations of SMS in children and adults. Brachycephaly, broad, flat face, synophrys, strabismus, downturned lip, prognathism, and malformed pinnae are noticeable. (From Greenberg et al., 1996. *Am. J. Med. Genet.* 62:247–254. Copyright © 1996 John Wiley & Sons, Inc. Reprinted by permission of Wiley-Liss, Inc.)

REFERENCES

Greenberg F, Guzzetta V, Montes de Oca-Luna R, Magenis RE, Smith AC, Richter SF, Kondo I, Dobyns WB, Patel PI, Lupski JR. 1991. Molecular analysis of the Smith–Magenis syndrome: a possible contiguous-gene syndrome associated with del(17)(p11.2). *Am. J. Hum. Genet.* 49:1207–1218.

Greenberg F, Lewis RA, Potocki L, Glaze D, Parke J, Killian J, Murphy MA, Williamson D, Brown F, Dutton R, McCluggage C, Friedman E, Sulek M, Lupski JR. 1996. Multi-disciplinary clinical study of Smith–Magenis syndrome (deletion 17p11.2). *Am. J. Med. Genet.* 62:247–254.

Kondo I, Matsuura S, Kuwajima K, Tokashiki M, Izumikawa Y, Naritomi K, Niikawa N, Kajii T. 1991. Diagnostic hand anomalies in Smith–Magenis syndrome: four new patients with del(17)(p11.2p11.2). *Am. J. Med. Genet.* 41:225–229.

Natacci F, Corrado L, Pierri M, Rossetti M, Zuccarini C, Riva P, Miozzo M, Larizza L. 2000. Patient with large 17p11.2 deletion presenting with Smith–Magenis syndrome and Joubert syndrome phenotype. *Am. J. Med. Genet.* 95:467–472.

Park JP, Moeschler JB, Davies WS, Patel PI, Mohandas TK. 1998. Smith–Magenis syndrome resulting from a de novo direct insertion of proximal 17q into 17p11.2. *Am. J. Med. Genet.* 77:23–27.

Smith AC, McGavran L, Robinson J, Waldstein G, Macfarlane J, Zonona J, Reiss J, Lahr M, Allen L, Magenis E. 1986. Interstitial deletion of (17)(p11.2p11.2) in nine patients. *Am. J. Med. Genet.* 24:393–414.

Zori RT, Lupski JR, Heju Z, Greenberg F, Killian JM, Gray BA, Driscoll DJ, Patel PI, Zackowski JL. 1993. Clinical, cytogenetic, and molecular evidence for an infant with Smith–Magenis syndrome born from a mother having a mosaic 17p11.2p12 deletion. *Am. J. Med. Genet.* 47:504–511.

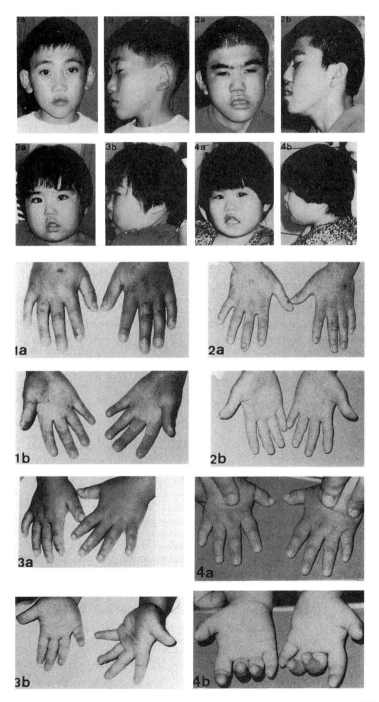

Facial appearance and limb manifestations of SMS in four Japanese patients aged 2 to 17 years old. (From Kondo et al., 1991. *Am. J. Med. Genet.* 41:225–229. Copyright © 1991 John Wiley & Sons, Inc. Reprinted by permission of Wiley-Liss, Inc.)

CHROMOSOME 17p13 MONOSOMY
Miller–Dieker Syndrome

Miller–Dieker syndrome is associated with microdeletions within bands 17p13. The phenotype includes characteristic craniofacial appearance and type I lissencephaly, seizures, and other neurological abnormalities.

MAIN FEATURES: Lissencephaly, high forehead, vertical furrows over forehead

ABNORMALITIES

Craniofacies: Wide, prominent forehead, with vertical deep furrows, bitemporal hollowing, short nose, prominent upper lip and small jaw, broad nasal bridge, epicanthal folds, low-set, malformed ears, and high-arched palate

Limbs: Deep palmar creases are seen in about two-thirds of the cases. Transverse palmar creases, clinodactyly, and flexion contractures are seen in 25–40% of the patients.

Other: Lissencephaly is always present. Hypoplasia of the corpus callosum, midline calcification, and cavum septum pellucidum are other common features. Congenital heart defects are seen in about 25% of the patients. Sacral dimple and genital anomaly in males are other common manifestations.

CLINICAL COURSE: Severe to profound mental retardation is consistently present. Life span is reduced. Most reported cases are infants.

CYTOGENETICS: The combined use of high-resolution cytogenetics and fluorescence in situ hybridization (FISH) are necessary to establish a diagnosis of clinically suspected cases of Miller–Dieker syndrome. About 80% of the cases are due to de novo mutation. Translocations, inversions, and cryptic translocation are known. Parents and other appropriate relatives of an index case should be studied for complete genetic diagnosis and counseling. Prenatal diagnosis is possible by chorionic villus sampling (CVS), amniocentesis, and FISH analysis.

REFERENCES

Dobyns WB, Curry CJ, Hoyme HE, Turlington L, Ledbetter DH. 1991. Clinical and molecular diagnosis of Miller–Dieker syndrome. *Am. J. Hum. Genet.* 48:584–594.

Kuwano A, Ledbetter SA, Dobyns WB, Emanuel BS, Ledbetter DH. 1991. Detection of deletions and cryptic translocations in Miller–Dieker syndrome by in situ hybridization. *Am. J. Hum. Genet.* 49:707–714.

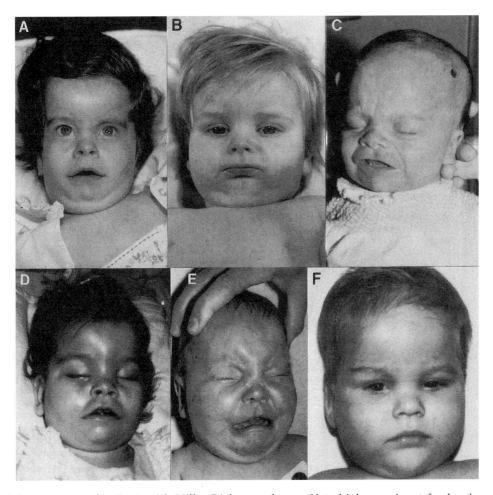

Facial appearance of patients with Miller-Dieker syndrome. Note high prominent forehead, vertical furrows, broad nasal bridge, short nose, prominent upper lip, wide mouth, and small jaw. Patients B and F had normal chromosomes and manifested milder features. (From Dobyns et al., 1991. *Am. J. Hum. Genet.* 48:584–594. Copyright © 1991 John Wiley & Sons, Inc. Reprinted by permission of Wiley-Liss, Inc.)

Ledbetter SA, Kuwano A, Dobyns WB, Ledbetter DH. 1992. Microdeletions of chromosome 17p13 as a cause of isolated lissencephaly. *Am. J. Hum. Genet.* 50:182–189.

Pilz DT, Dalton A, Long A, Jaspan T, Maltby EL, Quarrell OW. 1995. Detecting deletions in the critical region for lissencephaly on 17p13.3 using fluorescent in situ hybridisation and a PCR assay identifying a dinucleotide repeat polymorphism. *J. Med. Genet.* 32:275–278.

Schwartz CE, Johnson JP, Holycross B, Mandeville TM, Sears TS, Graul EA, Carey JC, Schroer RJ, Phelan MC, Szollar J, et al. 1988. Detection of submicroscopic deletions in band 17p13 in patients with the Miller–Dieker syndrome. *Am. J. Hum. Genet.* 43:597–604.

Sharief N, Craze J, Summers D, Butler L, Wood CB. 1991. Miller–Dieker syndrome with ring chromosome 17. *Arch. Dis. Child.* 66:710–712.

Yang SP, Bidichandani SI, Figuera LE, Juyal RC, Saxon PJ, Baldini A, Patel PI. 1997. Molecular analysis of deletion (17)(p11.2p11.2) in a family segregating a 17p paracentric inversion: implications for carriers of paracentric inversions. *Am. J. Hum. Genet.* 60:1184–1193.

CHROMOSOME 17q PARTIAL TRISOMY

At least 30 cases of partial trisomy 17q have been published. Sarri et al. (1997) have provided a comprehensive review.

MAIN FEATURES: Psychomotor retardation, microcephaly, frontal bossing, broad, flat nasal bridge, malformed ears

GENERAL CHARACTERISTICS: Short stature and developmental delay are always present. Craniofacial and limb anomalies are characteristic. Cardiac and central nervous system (CNS) anomalies are also frequent.

ABNORMALITIES

Craniofacies: The anomalies noted and the number of patients in whom specific mention was made of their presence or absence are microcephaly (16 of 18), frontal bossing (18 of 20), bitemporal narrowing (17 of 19), cranial/facial asymmetry (14 of 20), hypertelorism and broad nasal bridge (12 of 15), flat nasal bridge (16 of 20), wide mouth (10 of 15), thin upper lip (11 of 20), micrognathia (18 of 23), low-set ears (18 of 20), and malformed ears (6 of 6).

Limbs: Polydactyly of hands and feet, syndactyly of fingers as well as toes was present in 50% of the cases. Proximal shortening of the limbs (rhizomelia) was noted in 16 of 20 patients. Hyperlaxity of the limb joints was present in 9 of 15 cases reported.

Other: Short, webbed neck, low posterior hairline, widely spaced nipples were present in >70% of the patients. Anomalies of the CNS, heart, kidneys, and gastrointestinal tract were also frequently noted (>50%).

CLINICAL COURSE: Most cases are infants and children. At least two have survived to adulthood.

CYTOGENETICS: Most cases are due to malsegregation of balanced translocations present in one of the parents. Three were associated with pericentric inversions. One case each of tandem direct duplication and inverted duplication and two cases of X-autosome translocation have allowed comparisons of "pure 17q duplications" with those associated with partial monosomies of other chromosomes. Specific genotype–karyotype correlations with proximal versus distal duplication have not emerged.

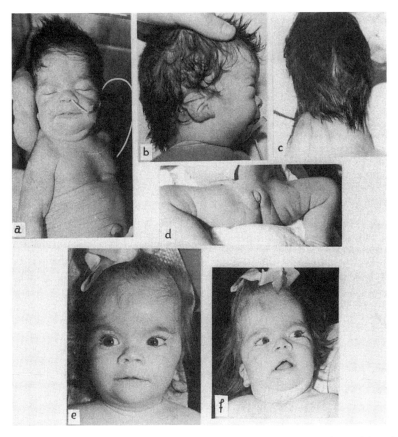

Multiple views of the craniofacial appearance and clitoris hypertrophy of a child with dup(17)(q22qter) at 10 days (a–d) and at 1 year and 1 month (e,f). (From Sarri et al., 1997. *Am. J. Med. Genet.* 70:87–94. Copyright © 1997 John Wiley & Sons, Inc. Reprinted by permission of Wiley-Liss, Inc.)

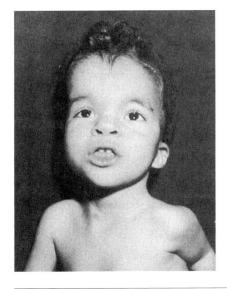

A boy 1 year and 7 months of age in whom duplication (17)(q23qter) was associated with del(12)(q24qter). (From Naccache et al., 1984. *Am. J. Med. Genet.* 17:633–639. Copyright © 1984 John Wiley & Sons, Inc. Reprinted by permission of Wiley-Liss, Inc.)

REFERENCES

Bridge J, Sanger W, Mosher G, Buehler B, Hearty C, Olney A, Fordyce R. 1985. Partial duplication of distal 17q. *Am. J. Med. Genet.* 22:229–235.

King PA, Ghosh A, Tang M. 1991. Mosaic partial trisomy 17q2. *J. Med. Genet.* 28:641–643.

Naccache NF, Vianna-Morgante AM, Richieri-Costa A. 1984. Brief clinical report: duplication of distal 17q: report of an observation. *Am. J. Med. Genet.* 17:633–639.

Ohdo S, Madokoro H, Sonoda T, Ohba K. 1989. Sibs lacking characteristic features of duplication of distal 17q. *J. Med. Genet.* 26:465–468.

Sarri C, Gyftodimou J, Avramopoulos D, Grigoriadou M, Pedersen W, Pandelia E, Pangalos C, Abazis D, Kitsos G, Vassilopoulos D, Brondum-Nielsen K, Petersen MB. 1997. Partial trisomy 17q22-qter and partial monosomy Xq27-qter in a girl with a de novo unbalanced translocation due to a postzygotic error: case report and review of the literature on partial trisomy 17qter. *Am. J. Med. Genet.* 70:87–94.

Shimizu T, Ikeuchi T, Shinohara T, Ohba S, Miyaguchi H, Akiyama T, Shibata T. 1988. Distal trisomy of chromosome 17q due to inverted tandem duplication. *Clin. Genet.* 33:311–314.

CHROMOSOME 17q PARTIAL MONOSOMY

There are at least seven published cases of 17q interstitial deletions with overlapping breakpoints. Their clinical description and photographs are the basis for this summary.

ABNORMALITIES

Craniofacies: Microcephaly, brachycephaly, round face, upward-slanted palpebral fissures, and mild or questionable micrognathia were present in at least four of the seven patients. Ears were not malformed or posteriorly rotated. No cleft lip or palate was present in any patient except for one with a bifid uvula. Hypertelorism was present in 3 of the 7 cases.

Limbs: Proximal placement of the thumbs (6 of 7) and symphalangism (5 of 7) were a somewhat unique combination of findings that may be of diagnostic value.

Other: Developmental delay was present in all patients and varied from mild to moderate when assessment was possible. Growth failure, poor feeding, irritability during infancy, abnormal gait reminiscent of Angelman syndrome (in one case) have been noted. Malformations have included T-E fistula (2 cases), congenital heart defects (3 cases) and 2 cases each with undescended testes and inguinal hernia.

CLINICAL COURSE: Most cases have been infants or children. Life expectancy is unknown.

CYTOGENETICS: Deletion breakpoints have included 17q21.3 to 17q24.3. The smallest deletion involving only bands 17q23.1q23.3 showed a phenotype not too different from the others, suggesting a major role for 17q23 in the causation of the phenotype.

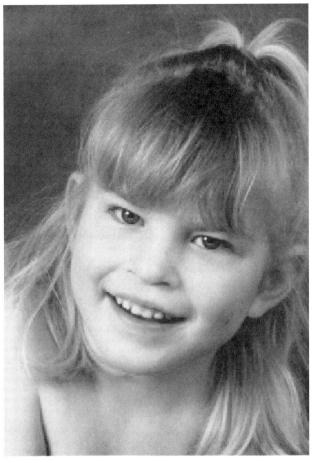

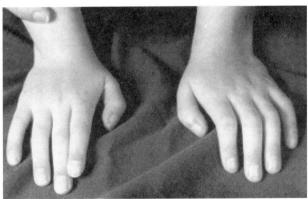

Facial appearance and hands of a girl 4 years and 6 months of age. Note proximally placed thumbs and symphalangism of digits 2–5. (From Mickelson et al., 1997. *Am. J. Med. Genet.* 71:275–279. Copyright © 1997 John Wiley & Sons, Inc. Reprinted by permission of Wiley-Liss, Inc.)

REFERENCES

Dallapiccola B, Mingarelli R, Digilio C, Obregon MG, Giannotti A. 1993. Interstitial deletion del(17)(q21.3q23 or 24.2) syndrome. *Clin. Genet.* 43:54–55.

Khalifa MM, MacLeod PM, Duncan AM. 1993. Additional case of de novo interstitial deletion del(17)(q21.3q23) and expansion of the phenotype. *Clin. Genet.* 44:258–261.

Levin ML, Shaffer LG, Lewis RAp6, Gresik MV, Lupski JR. 1995. Unique de novo interstitial deletion of chromosome 17, del(17)(q23.2q24.3) in a female newborn with multiple congenital anomalies. *Am. J. Med. Genet.* 55:30–32.

Mickelson EC, Robinson WP, Hrynchak MA, Lewis ME. 1997. Novel case of del(17)(q23.1q23.3) further highlights a recognizable phenotype involving deletions of chromosome (17)(q21q24). *Am. J. Med. Genet.* 71:275–279.

Park JP, Moeschler JB, Berg SZ, Bauer RM, Wurster-Hill DH. 1992. A unique de novo interstitial deletion del(17)(q2l.3q23) in a phenotypically abnormal infant. *Clin. Genet.* 41:54–56.

Thomas JA, Manchester DK, Prescott KE, Milner R, McGavran L, Cohen MM Jr. 1996. Hunter-McAlpine craniosynostosis phenotype associated with skeletal anomalies and interstitial deletion of chromosome 17q. *Am. J. Med. Genet.* 62:372–375.

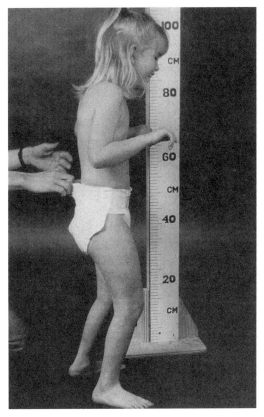

Note broad-based, unsteady gait. (From Mickelson et al., 1997. *Am. J. Med. Genet.* 71:275–279. Copyright © 1997 John Wiley & Sons, Inc. Reprinted by permission of Wiley-Liss, Inc.)

CHROMOSOME 18 TRISOMY

Trisomy 18, known as a distinctive syndrome since 1960, is a relatively common and clinically recognizable pattern of malformation with an estimated incidence of about 1:5000 to 1:8000 newborns. Trisomy 18 is highly lethal to fetuses as well as newborns. More than 100 malformations have been noted in patients with trisomy 18, the most frequent of which are summarized here.

MAIN FEATURES: Intrauterine growth retardation, small palpebral fissures, small mouth, rocker-bottom feet, characteristic hand posture.

GENERAL CHARACTERISTICS: Intrauterine growth retardation is prominent with a mean birth weight estimated to be 2240 gm. Both premature and postmature births are common. Maternal-age effect is known, but advanced maternal age is not associated with most trisomy 18 births. Pregnancy complications include polyhydramnios, small placenta, and single umbilical artery.

ABNORMALITIES

Craniofacies: Facial features are distinctive and include small palpebral fissures, wide, high forehead, large fontanelle, prominent occiput, small mouth, receding chin, and low-set, posteriorly rotated ears with pointed upper helix. A trisomy 18 scoring system has been published (Marion et al., 1988). Corneal clouding, cataracts, microphthalmia may be seen, but cleft lip or palate are less common than in trisomy 13. Choanal stenosis or atresia may be present.

Genitourinary: Horseshoe kidney, ectopic kidney, hydronephrosis, duplication of the ureter, undescended testes, and hypospadias.

Limbs: The characteristic hand posture of trisomy 18 infants consists of overlapping of second finger over third and fifth over the fourth with thumbs in apposition with the index fingers. Rocker-bottom feet and a proximally implanted, short hallux are quite typical. Radial defects of the upper limb are common.

Organs: Congenital heart defects, mostly ventricular and atrial septal defects, are quite common. Gastrointestinal anomalies include pyloric stenosis, Meckel's diverticulum, and ectopic pancreas. Diaphragmatic hypoplasia with eventration, diaphragmatic hernia, and abnormal segmentation of the lung may be seen.

Other: Musculoskeletal features include generalized muscle hypoplasia, hypertonicity, hip dysplasia, narrow pelvis, and hemivertebrae.

Central nervous system: Central nervous system (CNS) malformations are not as common as in trisomy 13; however, neural tube closure defects are associated with trisomy 18. A feeble cry, poor suck, central apnea, and seizures occur frequently and contribute to early demise of infants with trisomy 18.

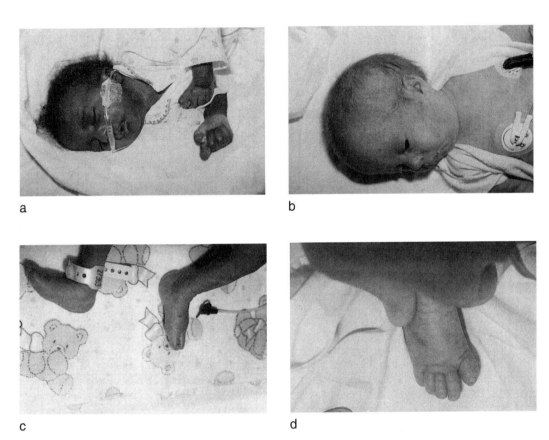

Infants with trisomy 18 showing dolichocephaly, high, wide forehead, micrognathia, small mouth, low-set, posteriorly rotated ears, high nasal bridge, small palpebral fissure (a,b), and the characteristic hand posture (a). Rocker-bottom feet (c) and short great toe (d) are also part of the phenotype.

CLINICAL COURSE: Trisomy 18 is highly lethal during infancy with only 5–10% of the patients living through their first year of life. Growth and development show severe to profound impairment. Rare survivors to adulthood are known and have minimal cognitive function. This poor prognosis has led many medical professionals and ethicists to recommend only comfort care and withholding of major surgical intervention or life-prolonging intensive care for infants with trisomy 18. There are exceptionally rare instances of individuals with normal intelligence and trisomy 18 found in late childhood or adulthood. They are usually mosaic for a normal cell line with trisomy 18 confined to a minor proportion of the cells. Survival and long-term prognosis have been reviewed by Baty et al. (1994).

CYTOGENETICS: Most patients have full trisomy 18 resulting from meiotic nondisjunction. Maternal age is a risk factor. Partial trisomies and mosaicism may dilute the phenotypic effects. A critical region for major manifestations of trisomy 18 has not been defined.

PRENATAL DIAGNOSIS: Prenatal detection of trisomy 18 is possible by chromosomal studies of amniotic fluid cells and chorionic villus samples. Maternal serum markers for trisomy 18 include alpha-fetoprotein, human chorionic gonadotropin, and unconjugated estriol. Fetal sonography also can identify a number fetal anomalies associated with trisomy 18, including growth restriction, nuchal transluscency, choroid plexus cysts, two-vessel cord, and a variety of cardiac, renal, diaphragmatic, CNS, or limb anomalies.

REFERENCES

Baty BJ, Blackburn BL, Carey JC. 1994. Natural history of trisomy 18 and trisomy 13: I. Growth, physical assessment, medical histories, survival, and recurrence risk. *Am. J. Med. Genet.* 49:175–188.

Baty BJ, Jorde LB, Blackburn BL, Carey JC. 1994. Natural history of trisomy 18 and trisomy 13: II. Psychomotor development. *Am. J. Med. Genet.* 49:189–194.

Carter PE, Pearn JH, Bell J, Martin N, Anderson NG. 1985. Survival in trisomy 18. Life tables for use in genetic counselling and clinical paediatrics. *Clin. Genet.* 27:59–61.

Ginsberg N, Cadkin A, Pergament E, Verlinsky Y. 1990. Ultrasonographic detection of the second-trimester fetus with trisomy 18 and trisomy 21. *Am. J. Obstet. Gynecol.* 163:1186–1190.

Marion RW, Chitayat D, Hutcheon RG, Neidich JA, Zackai EH, Singer LP, Warman M. 1988. Trisomy 18 score: a rapid, reliable diagnostic test for trisomy 18. *J. Pediatr.* 113:45–48.

Mucke J, Trautmann U, Sandig KR, Theile H. 1982. The crucial band for phenotype of trisomy 18. *Hum. Genet.* 60:205.

Palomaki GE, Haddow JE, Knight GJ, Wald NJ, Kennard A, Canick JA, Saller DN Jr, Blitzer MG, Dickerman LH, Fisher R. 1995. Risk-based prenatal screening for trisomy 18 using alpha-fetoprotein, unconjugated oestriol and human chorionic gonadotropin. *Prenat. Diagn.* 15:713–723.

Snijders RJ, Shawa L, Nicolaides K. 1994. Fetal choroid plexus cysts and trisomy 18: assessment of risk based on ultrasound findings and maternal age. *Prenat. Diagn.* 14:1119–1127.

Wilson GN, Heller KB, Elterman RD, Schneider NR. 1990. Partial trisomy 18 with minimal anomalies: lack of correspondence between phenotypic manifestations and triplicated loci along chromosome 18. *Am. J. Med. Genet.* 36:506–510.

Wolff DJ, Schwartz MF, Cohen MM, Schwartz S. 1993. Precise mapping of a de novo duplication 18(q21 → q22) utilizing cytogenetic, biochemical, and molecular techniques. *Am. J. Med. Genet.* 46:520–523.

CHROMOSOME 18p PARTIAL MONOSOMY

The 18p monosomy syndrome was first described by deGrouchy et al. in 1963. More than 100 cases had been identified by the 1980s, indicating that the syndrome was common. However, no good estimates of its incidence or prevalence are available.

MAIN FEATURES: Short stature, microcephaly, psychomotor retardation

GENERAL CHARACTERISTICS: Short stature is considered the most consistent finding. Failure to thrive and global developmental delay also are quite common.

ABNORMALITIES

Craniofacies: Microcephaly, flat midface, round face, hypertelorism, ptosis, epicanthal folds are reported in 50% of the patients. Cleft palate, carp-shaped mouth, microretrognathia, large, protruding ears are somewhat less common. However, facial dysmorphism can be quite subtle, and girls whose main feature is only short stature may be suspected to have the Turner syndrome.

Organs: Central nervous system (CNS) malformations ranging from arrhinencephaly/holoprosencephaly sequence to what some consider its minimal manifestation—hypertelorism—are part of this syndrome. The empty-sella syndrome with pituitary dysfunction and associated with the single central maxillary incisor have been found on several occasions. Good response to growth hormone therapy has been documented. Gonadal dysgenesis has been reported. Congenital heart defects have been rarely reported.

CLINICAL COURSE: Except for those born with the severe midline CNS defects there are no serious malformations or life-threatening symptoms associated with the 18p deletion syndrome. Survival to adulthood is common. Life expectancy is unknown. Immunoglobulin A (IgA) deficiency reported in some patients has not presented functional immunological difficulties.

CYTOGENETICS: Most cases occur de novo. Features of 18p deletion can be associated with ring (18) syndrome. Parent-to-child transmission of 18p deletion has been reported. Malsegregation of a partial balanced structural abnormality should be sought. Prenatal diagnosis has been made by amniocentesis.

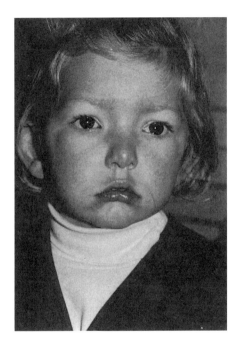

Three-year-old girl with 18p deletion identified because of short stature, congenital lymphedema, coarctation of the aorta. Note minimal facial dysmorphism. (From Telvi et al., 1995. *Am. J. Med. Genet.* 57:598–600. Copyright © 1995 John Wiley & Sons, Inc. Reprinted by permission of Wiley-Liss, Inc.)

REFERENCES

Aughton DJ, AlSaadi AA, Transue DJ. 1991. Single maxillary central incisor in a girl with del(18p) syndrome. *J. Med. Genet.* 28:530–532.

DeGrouchy J, Lamy M, Thieffry S, Arthuis M, Salmon C. 1963. Dysmorphic complexe avec oligophrenie: deletion des bras courts d'un chromosome 17–18. *C.R. Acad. Sci.* 256:1028–1029.

Dolan LM, Willson K, Wilson WG. 1981. 18p-syndrome with a single central maxillary incisor. *J. Med. Genet.* 18:396–398.

Faust J, Habedank M, Nieuwenhuijsen C. 1976. The 18p-syndrome. Report of four cases. *Eur. J. Pediatr.* 123:59–66.

Fitzgerald MG. 1974. The 18p-syndrome: a case report and brief review of the literature. *Aust. Paediatr. J.* 10:373–377.

Kuchle M, Kraus J, Rummelt C, Naumann GO. 1991. Synophthalmia and holoprosencephaly in chromosome 18p deletion defect. *Arch. Ophthalmol.* 109:136–137.

Schinzel A, Schmid W, Luscher U, Nater M, Brook C, Steinmann B. 1974. Structural aberrations of chromosome 18. I. The 18p-syndrome. *Arch. Genet.* 47:1–15.

Schober E, Scheibenreiter S, Frisch H. 1995. 18p monosomy with GH-deficiency and empty sella: good response to GH-treatment. *Clin. Genet.* 47:254–256.

Taine L, Goizet C, Wen ZQ, Chateil JF, Battin J, Saura R, Lacombe D. 1997. 18p monosomy with midline defects and a de novo satellite identified by FISH. *Ann. Genet.* 40:158–163.

Telvi L, Bernheim A, Ion A, Fouquet F, Le Bouc Y, Chaussain JL. 1995. Gonadal dysgenesis in del(18p) syndrome. *Am. J. Med. Genet.* 57:598–600.

Tsukahara M, Imaizumi K, Fujita K, Tateishi H, Uchida M. 2001. Familial Del(18p) syndrome. *Am. J. Med. Genet.* 99:67–69.

Velagaleti GV, Harris S, Carpenter NJ, Coldwell J, Say B. 1996. Familial deletion of chromosome 18(p11.2). *Ann. Genet.* 39:201–204.

CHROMOSOME 18q PARTIAL MONOSOMY

Originally described by deGrouchy et al. (1964), the 18q monosomy syndrome is among the most common autosomal segmental aneusomies. More than 100 cases have been reported. The estimated incidence is 1 in 40,000 live births. Cody et al. (1999) provided a detailed study of 42 patients including phenotype–karyotype correlations.

MAIN FEATURES: Microcephaly, turricephaly, deep-set eyes, carp-shaped mouth, broad philtrum.

GENERAL CHARACTERISTICS: Short stature is usually postnatal in onset. Birth weight has been generally in the normal range.

ABNORMALITIES

Craniofacies: Microcephaly, tall forehead, deep-set eyes, broad nasal bridge, and carp-shaped mouth with broad philtrum are common. Ear anomalies have included prominent antihelix and antitragus and atretic canals. Highly arched palate, cleft palate with or without cleft lip, submucous cleft palate, and bifid uvula have been found in <10% of the patients. Microphthalmia and cataracts are occasionally seen.

Genitourinary: Hypoplasia of the labia or scrotum (30–50%), micropenis (10–30%), and cryptorchidism (50–80%) has been reported (Strathdee et al., 1995).

Limbs: Small hands and feet, long, tapering digits, fleshy fingertips, short metacarpals and thumb are common. Dermatoglyphic characteristics include a high frequency of digital whorls, distal axial triradius, and simian creases. Feet show talipes equinovarus.

Organs: Organ malformations are rare. Occasionally horseshoe-shaped kidney, minor skeletal anomalies, and heart malformation may occur. However, absence of major internal malformation is a remarkable aspect of this syndrome.

Other: Moderate to severe mental retardation is usually present. Aggressive behavior and autistic tendencies have been reported. Movement disorders such as ataxia, dysmetria, choreoathetosis, and hypotonia have been associated with 18q partial monosomy. Seizures may be seen. Brain MRI studies have shown abnormalities of myelination, cerebellar hypoplasia, and hydrocephalus. Decreased or absent serum immunoglobulin A levels have been reported in about 25% of the patients. Isolated instances of growth hormone deficiency, Rett syndrome, serum carnosinase deficiency, and celiac disease have been reported. 18q monosomy has been reported in fetuses, infants, children and adults.

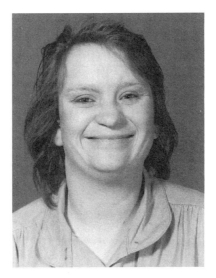

Adult female with 18q interstitial deletion showing minimal facial asymmetry, upward-slanting palpebral fissures. (From Miller et al., 1990. *Am. J. Med. Genet.* 37:128–132. Copyright © 1990 John Wiley & Sons, Inc. Reprinted by permission of Wiley-Liss, Inc.)

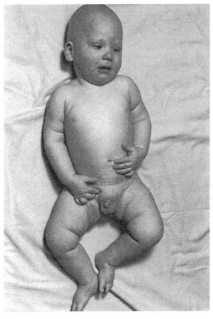
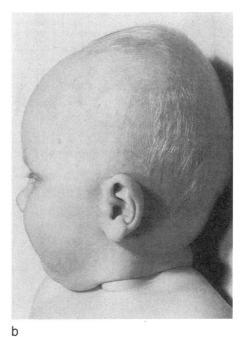

a   b

Son of adult female patient at 10 months showing small pinnae with prominent antihelix and redundant skin around the neck (a,b). (From Miller et al., 1990. *Am. J. Med. Genet.* 37:128–132. Copyright © 1990 John Wiley & Sons, Inc. Reprinted by permission of Wiley-Liss, Inc.)

CLINICAL COURSE: No reliable estimates are available for life expectancy. Absence of serious organ system malformation suggests that prolonged survival is likely for most patients.

CYTOGENETICS: Most deletions are terminal, but interstitial deletions are also common. Clinical correlations with karyotypic and molecular findings show that the common features of the 18q monosomy syndrome are associated with deletion of bands 18q12.1q21.1. Mother-to-child transmission of an interstitial deletion has been recorded. Parental origin studies have not found parent-of-origin effects.

REFERENCES

Brkanac Z, Cody JD, Leach RJ, DuPont BR. 1998. Identification of cryptic rearrangements in patients with 18q-deletion syndrome. *Am. J. Hum. Genet.* 62:1500–1506.

Cody JD, Ghidoni PD, DuPont BR, Hale DE, Hilsenbeck SG, Stratton RF, Hoffman DS, Muller S, Schaub RL, Leach RJ, Kaye CI. 1999. Congenital anomalies and anthropometry of 42 individuals with deletions of chromosome 18q. *Am. J. Med. Genet.* 85:455–462.

DeGrouchy J, Roper P, Salmon C. 1964. Deletion partiele des bras longs du chromosome 18. *Pathol. Biol. (Paris)* 12:579–582.

Ghidoni PD, Hale DE, Cody JD, Gay CT, Thompson NM, McClure EB, Danney MM, Leach RJ, Kaye CI. 1997. Growth hormone deficiency associated in the 18q deletion syndrome. *Am. J. Med. Genet.* 69:7–12.

Kline AD, White ME, Wapner R, Rojas K, Biesecker LG, Kamholz J, Zackai EH, Muenke M, Scott CI Jr, Overhauser J. 1993. Molecular analysis of the 18q-syndrome—and correlation with phenotype. *Am. J. Hum. Genet.* 52:895–906.

Lipschutz W, Cadranel S, Lipschutz B, Martin L, Clees N, Martin JJ, Wauters JG, Coucke P, Willems P. 1999. 18q-syndrome with coeliac disease. *Eur. J. Pediatr.* 158:528.

Miller G, Mowrey PN, Hopper KD, Frankel CA, Ladda RL. 1990. Neurologic manifestations in 18q-syndrome. *Am. J. Med. Genet.* 37:128–132.

Seshadri K, Wallerstein R, Burack G. 1992. 18q-chromosomal abnormality in a phenotypically normal 2 1/2-year-old male with autism. *Dev. Med. Child Neurol.* 34:1005–1009.

Strathdee G, Zackai EH, Shapiro R, Kamholz J, Overhauser J. 1995. Analysis of clinical variation seen in patients with 18q terminal deletions. *Am. J. Med. Genet.* 59:476–483.

Wilson MG, Towner JW, Forsman I, Siris E. 1979. Syndromes associated with deletion of the long arm of chromosome 18[del(18q)]. *Am. J. Med. Genet.* 3:155–174.

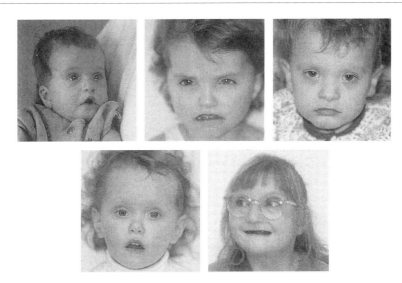

Facies of five children with 18q deletions. (From Cody et al., 1999. *Am. J. Med. Genet.* 85:455–462. Copyright © 1999 John Wiley & Sons, Inc. Reprinted by permission of Wiley-Liss, Inc.)

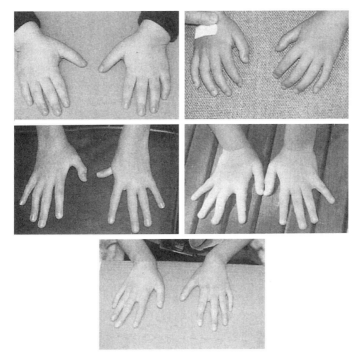

Hands of five 18q deletion patients demonstrating slender, tapering fingers, proximally placed anomalous thumbs, and fifth-finger clinodactyly. (From Cody et al., 1999. *Am. J. Med. Genet.* 85:455–462. Copyright © 1999 John Wiley & Sons, Inc. Reprinted by permission of Wiley-Liss, Inc.)

CHROMOSOME 19q PARTIAL TRISOMY

Duplications of the long arm of chromosome 19 have been described in at least 15 live-born individuals and a second-trimester fetus.

MAIN FEATURES: Growth retardation, microcephaly, downward slanting palpebral fissures down-turned corners of the mouth

GENERAL CHARACTERISTICS: Growth retardation, prenatal as well as postnatal, is almost always present (92%). Psychomotor developmental delay or mental retardation was observed in all live-born cases old enough to be assessed.

ABNORMALITIES

Craniofacies: Microcephaly was present in 9 of 13 cases. Wide anterior fontanelle, telecanthus, ptosis, downward-slanted palpebral fissures, flat face, short nose, short philtrum, downturned corners of the mouth, and abnormal ears were other features noted in >75% of the patients.

Limbs: Clinodactyly and brachydactyly were present in 50% of the patients. Simian crease, increased space between toes, flexion contractures, and congenital hip dysplasia were reported in <25% of the cases

Other: Short, thick neck with excessive nuchal skin was seen in virtually all live-born infants with 19q duplication. Interestingly, the one fetus diagnosed by chorionic villus sampling (CVS) in first trimester had a cystic hygroma. Congenital heart defects, genitourinary, and gastrointestinal malformations have been reported.

CLINICAL COURSE: The reported cases were 76 days to 25 years old at the time of report. Hypotonia and severe psychomotor retardation were present in all the older children and one adult patient.

CYTOGENETICS: The earliest reports mostly included partial trisomy 19q due to malsegregation of translocations. More recently, cases of "pure partial 19q" trisomy have been identified by fluorescence in situ hybridization (FISH) and high-resolution cytogenetics. Phenotype–karyotype correlations between the various duplicated segments have not been possible.

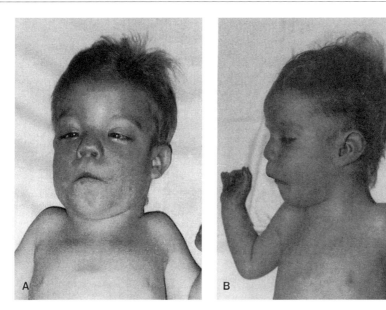

Profoundly retarded infant at 1 year and 6 months trisomic for 19q13.3qter secondary to t(19;22)(q13.3;pll) mat. (From Boyd et al., 1992. *Am. J. Med. Genet.* 42:326–330. Copyright © 1992 John Wiley & Sons, Inc. Reprinted by permission of Wiley-Liss, Inc.)

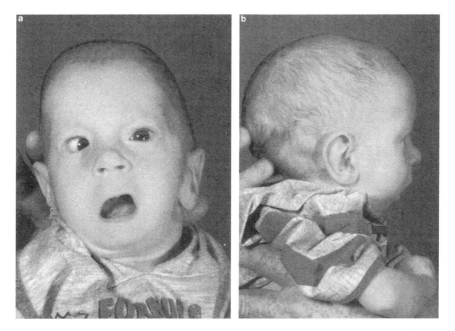

Male 1 year and 6 months with de novo duplication of bands 19q13.3q13.4 identified by high-resolution cytogenetics and FISH. (From Bhat et al., 2000. *Am. J. Med. Genet.* 91:201–203. Copyright © 2000 John Wiley & Sons, Inc. Reprinted by permission of Wiley-Liss, Inc.)

REFERENCES

Bhat M, Morrison PJ, Getty A, McManus D, Tubman R, Nevin NC. 2000. First clinical case of small de novo duplication of 19q(13.3–13.4) confirmed by FISH. *Am. J. Med. Genet.* 91:201–203.

Boyd E, Grass FS, Parke JC, Knutson K, Stevenson RE. 1992. Duplication of distal 19q: clinical report and review. *Am. J. Med. Genet.* 42:326–330.

Cotter PD, McCurdy LD, Gershin IF, Babu A, Willner JP, Desnick RJ. 1997. Prenatal detection and molecular characterization of a de novo duplication of the distal long arm of chromosome 19. *Am. J. Med. Genet.* 71:325–328.

James C, Jauch A, Robson L, Watson N, Smith A. 1996. A 3 1/2 year old girl with distal trisomy 19q defined by FISH. *J. Med. Genet.* 33:795–797.

Lange M, Alfi OS. 1976. Trisomy 19q. *Ann. Genet.* 19:17–21.

Madokoro H, Ohdo S, Sonoda T, Kawaguchi K, Ohba K. 1988. Partial trisomy for 19q due to paternal 17/19 reciprocal translocation. *Jinrui. Idengaku. Zasshi.* 33:61–65.

Rivas F, Garcia-Cruz D, Rivera H, Plascencia ML, Gonzalez RM, Cantu JM. 1985. 19q distal trisomy due to a de novo (19;22)(q13.2;p11) translocation. *Ann. Genet.* 27:113–115.

Schmid W. 1979. Trisomy for the distal third of the long arm of chromosome 19 in brother and sister. *Hum. Genet.* 46:263–270.

Valerio D, Lavorgna F, Scalona M, Conte A. 1993. A new case of partial trisomy 19q(q13.2 → qter) owing to an unusual maternal translocation. *J. Med. Genet.* 30:697–699.

Zonana J, Brown MG, Magenis RE. 1982. Distal 19q duplication. *Hum. Genet.* 60:267–270.

RING CHROMOSOME 19

Clinical manifestations of ring chromosome 19 abnormality can vary from completely normal to profound mental retardation with minimal dysmorphism. As with other autosomal ring syndromes, the lack of a distinctive phenotype means that clinical diagnosis is not possible and prenatal detection of a case may present counseling dilemmas. The hypotheses put forth to account for the clinical variability of ring chromosome carriers include variability in the length of deleted segments, the variable presence of a normal cell line and the varying tissue distribution due to the inherent instability of ring chromosomes.

ABNORMALITIES

Craniofacies: Microcephaly, high forehead, high nasal bridge, low-set and posteriorly rotated ears, in-turned upper lip, hypertelorism, prominent philtrum, and micrognathia

Limbs: Digital hypoplasia, clubfoot, and joint contractures were seen in one patient.

Organs: Pulmonic stenosis, hypoplastic right ventricle, and coronary artery fistula

Other: Intrauterine and postnatal growth retardation and mild to profound developmental delay and mental retardation, absent speech and autistic behavior have been reported.

CYTOGENETICS: De novo as well as familial cases are known. Mosaicism is common as expected.

REFERENCES

Flejter WL, Finlinson D, Root S, Nguyen W, Brothman AR, Viskochil D. 1996. Familial ring (19) chromosome mosaicism: case report and review. *Am. J. Med. Genet.* 66:276–280.

Ghaffari SR, Boyd E, Connor JM, Jones AM, Tolmie J. 1998. Mosaic supernumerary ring chromosome 19 identified by comparative genomic hybridisation. *J. Med. Genet.* 35:836–840.

Gillessen-Kaesbach G, Ngo NT. 1990. Ring 19 mosaicism detected during prenatal diagnosis. *Prenat. Diagn.* 10:683–687.

Sybert VP, Bradley CM, Salk D. 1988. Mosaicism for ring 19: a case report. *Clin. Genet.* 34:382–385.

Uchida IA, Lin CC. 1972. Ring formation of chromosomes nos. 19 and 20. *Cytogenetics* 11:208–215.

Vaz I, Larkins SA, Norman A, Green SH. 1999. Mild developmental delay due to ring chromosome 19 mosaicism. *Dev. Med. Child Neurol.* 41:48–50.

Yung JF, Sobel DB, Hoo JJ. 1990. Origin of 46,XY/46,XY,r(19) mosaicism. *Am. J. Med. Genet.* 36:391–393.

CHROMOSOME 20p PARTIAL TRISOMY

More than 30 clinical observations have contributed to the definition of a consistent pattern of malformation attributable to 20p partial trisomy.

MAIN FEATURES: Developmental delay, normal growth, round face, coarse hair, large nostrils

GENERAL CHARACTERISTICS: Unlike most other autosomal chromosome imbalances, 20p trisomy is not associated with poor physical growth. Birth weight is usually normal. Postnatal growth is also normal. Some individuals have been large for their age. At least one patient with Sotos syndrome has been identified with 46,XY,dup(20)(p11.2p12.1)/46,XY mosaicism. Male:female ratio is close to one. Many adult patients are known.

ABNORMALITIES

Craniofacies: A round face, mongoloid slant to the palpebral fissures, hypertelorism, strabismus, and short nose are present in >50% of the patients. Coarse hair and large nostrils are somewhat unique features noted in 70% of the patients. Epicanthal folds were seen in 38% of the patients.

Limbs: Clinodactyly and other anomalies of fingers and toes were present in 30–40% of the patients.

Other: The high incidence of dental anomalies (78%), vertebral defects (75%), poor motor coordination (94%), and poor speech (95%) constitutes a somewhat unique pattern that might lead to a clinical suspicion of this syndrome. Congenital heart defects (38%), hypospadias (16%), and macro-orchidism are other reported anomalies. Isolated cases of thyroid carcinoma and Sotos syndrome have been reported.

CLINICAL COURSE: Survival to adulthood is known. Mental retardation is consistently present.

CYTOGENETICS: Most cases are inherited due to malsegregation of parental translocations. Maternal as well as paternal transmissions have occurred. Pure trisomy 20p due to mosaic duplication of 20p11.2p12.1 was found in a patient with Sotos syndrome.

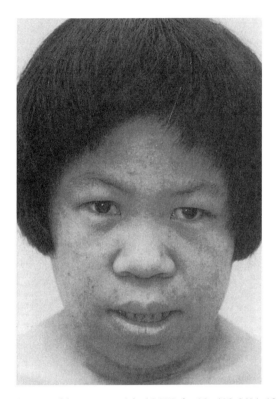

Facial appearance of an 18-year-old woman with 46,XX,der12,t(12;20)(p13.31; p11.2) pat. Note the wide philtrum, broad nose, flat nasal bridge, and prominant lower lip. (From Clark et al., 1993. *Am. J. Med. Genet.* 45:14–16. Copyright © 1993 John Wiley & Sons, Inc. Reprinted by permission of Wiley-Liss, Inc.)

REFERENCES

Balestrazzi P, Virdis R, Frassi C, Negri V, Rigoli E, Bernasconi S. 1984. "De Novo" trisomy 20p with macroorchidism in a prepuberal boy. *Ann. Genet.* 27:58–59.

Centerwall W, Francke U. 1977. Familial trisomy 20p. Five cases and two carriers in three generations a review. *Ann. Genet.* 20:77–83.

Chen H, Hoffman WH, Tyrkus M, Al Saadi A, Bawle E. 1983. Partial trisomy 20p syndrome and maternal mosaicism. *Ann. Genet.* 26:21–25.

Clark P, Jones KL, Freidenberg GR. 1993. Duplication (20p) in association with thyroid carcinoma. *Am. J. Med. Genet.* 45:14–16.

Grammatico P, Cupilari F, Di Rosa C, Falcolini M, Del Porto G. 1992. 20p duplication as a result of parental translocation: familial case report and a contribution to the clinical delineation of the syndrome. *Clin. Genet.* 41:285–289.

Faivre L, Viot G, Prieur M, Turleau C, Gosset P, Romana S, Munnich A, Vekemans M, Cormier-Daire V. 2000. Apparent sotos syndrome (cerebral gigantism) in a child with trisomy 20p11.2–p12.1 mosaicism. *Am. J. Med. Genet.* 91:273–276.

Funderburk SJ, Sparkes RS, Sparkes MC. 1983. Trisomy 20p due to a paternal reciprocal translocation. *Ann. Genet.* 26:94–97.

Karukaja S, Matsuyuki M, Shiotsuki Y, Kato H. 1982. A female infant with trisomy 20p. *Jpn. J. Hum. Genet.* 27:211–212.

Lurie IW, Rumyantseva NV, Zaletajev DV, Gurevich DB, Korotkova IA. 1985. Trisomy 20p: case report and genetic review. *J. Genet. Hum.* 33:67–75.

Schinzel A. 1980. Trisomy 20pter = to q11 in a malformed boy from a t(13;20)(p11;q11) translocation-carrier mother. *Hum. Genet.* 53:169–172.

CHROMOSOME 20p PARTIAL MONOSOMY

Only a small number of patients with deletion of the short arm of chromosome 20 have been reported. This summary is based on clinical descriptions of 10 patients who were considered to meet the diagnostic criteria for the Alagille syndrome (arteriohepatic dysplasia) associated with deletions of band 20p12 and 8 patients who did not meet the criteria. (Krantz et al., 1997; Teebi et al., 1992).

MAIN FEATURES: Developmental delay, failure to thrive, hypertelorism, long philtrum

GENERAL CHARACTERISTICS: Birth weight was normal or low for gestational age. There are 11 females and 7 males reported whose ages ranged from 6 months to 30 years at the time of the report. Developmental delay and failure to thrive are common.

ABNORMALITIES

Craniofacies: Flat facial profile, frontal bossing, wide open cranial sutures, hypertelorism, deeply set eyes, prominent, straight nose, posterior embryotoxon, pigmentary retinopathy, iris dysplasia, coloboma, epicanthal folds, long philtrum, short and wide neck with redundant nuchal skin fold

Other: Vertebral anomalies (hemivertebrae or butterfly vertebrae), renal anomalies, congenital heart defects, particularly pulmonary artery stenosis, liver disease (cholestatic jaundice, paucity of bile ducts) when present will probably lead to a clinical diagnosis of the Alagille syndrome. However, presence of developmental delay indicates a high likelihood of cytogenetically visible deletions within 20p.

Hirschsprung disease and autism have been reported in a patient with cytogenetically suspected deletion within 20p11.22p11.23. Molecular studies confirmed that the deletion did not overlap the putative Alagille locus.

CLINICAL COURSE: Survival to adulthood is known. Prognosis for survival may depend on severity of liver and heart defects.

CYTOGENETICS: Most cases of partial monosomy 20p were due to de novo mutations detected by high resolution cytogenetic and/or molecular studies. Alagille syndrome (arteriohepatic dysplasia), a dominantly inherited disorder characterized by intrahepatic paucity of bile ducts associated with cholestasis, mild facial dysmorphism, and congenital heart defects, is occasionally associated

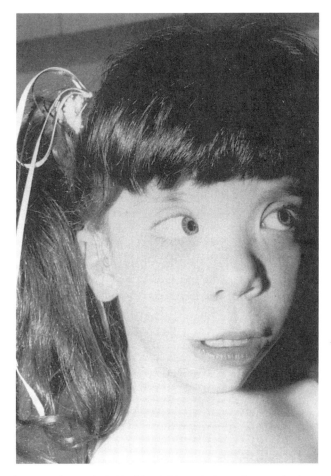

A girl at 6 years and 6 months with del(20)(p11.23pter). Note hypertelorism, maxillary hypoplasia, long philtrum, and upward-slanting corners of the mouth. (From Shohat et al., 1991. *Am. J. Med. Genet.* 39:56–63. Copyright © 1991 John Wiley & Sons, Inc. Reprinted by permission of Wiley-Liss, Inc.)

with cytogenetic or molecular deletions within band 20p12. Krantz et al. (1997) found 2 of 56 (3.6%) patients to have cytogenetically detectable 20p deletions. Molecular studies revealed only one additional case for a total of 3 out of 45 that underwent molecular analysis. They suggested that the Alagille syndrome may be caused by alteration of a single rather than multiple contiguous gene functions.

REFERENCES

Anad F, Burn J, Matthews D, Cross I, Davison BC, Mueller R, Sands M, Lillington DM, Eastham E. 1990. Alagille syndrome and deletion of 20p. *J. Med. Genet.* 27:729–737.

Byrne JL, Harrod MJ, Friedman JM, Howard-Peebles PN. 1986. del(20p) with manifestations of arteriohepatic dysplasia. *Am. J. Med. Genet.* 24:673–678.

Kalousek DK, Therien S. 1976. Deletion of the short arms of chromosome 20. *Hum. Genet.* 34:89–92.

Krantz ID, Rand EB, Genin A, Hunt P, Jones M, Louis AA, Graham JM Jr, Bhatt S, Piccoli DA, Spinner NB. 1997. Deletions of 20p12 in Alagille syndrome: frequency and molecular characterization. *Am. J. Med. Genet.* 70:80–86.

Michaelis RC, Skinner SA, Deason R, Skinner C, Moore CL, Phelan M. 1997. Intersitial deletion of 20p: new candidate region for Hirschsprung disease and autism? *Am. J. Med. Genet.* 71:298–304.

Shohat M, Herman V, Melmed S, Neufeld N, Schreck R, Pulst S, Graham JM Jr, Rimoin DL, Korenberg JR. 1991. Deletion of 20p11.23 → pter with normal growth hormone-releasing hormone genes. *Am. J. Med. Genet.* 39:56–63.

Silengo MC, Lopez Bell G, Biagioli M, Franceschini P. 1988. Partial deletion of the short arm of chromosome 20:46,XX,del(20)(p11)/46,XX mosaicism. *Clin. Genet.* 33:108–110.

Teebi AS, Murthy DS, Ismail EA, Redha AA. 1992. Alagille syndrome with de novo del(20)(p11.2). *Am. J. Med. Genet.* 42:35–38.

Vianna-Morgante AM, Richieri-Costa A, Rosenberg C. 1987. Deletion of the short arm of chromosome 20. *Clin. Genet.* 31:406–409.

RING CHROMOSOME 20

Ring chromosome 20 is associated with an intractable seizure disorder and characteristic electroencephalographic (EEG) abnormalities. At least 30 cases have been described since the initial description by Borgaonkar et al. (1976)

MAIN FEATURES: Seizures, developmental delay, normal growth, microcephaly, absence of malformation

GENERAL CHARACTERISTICS: Growth is usually normal. Developmental delay may not be evident for several years. Many patients were identified as adults often because of intractable epileptic seizures.

ABNORMALITIES

Craniofacial: No characteristic dysmorphism found

Limbs: No characteristic abnormalities noted

Malformations: No consistent malformations found

Central nervous system: Microcephaly, normal brain anatomy by neuroimaging, abnormal EEG. Non-convulsive status epilepticus (NCSE) may be a key feature of this syndrome

CLINICAL COURSE: Survival to adulthood is common. Mental retardation, behavioral disorder and intractable epilepsy are the major therapeutic issues.

CYTOGENETICS: Most cases have been sporadic. One instance of transmission from a clinically normal mother to two of her children has been recorded. Mosaicism is common and variable. There does not appear to be a correlation between percentage of r(20) cells and severity of the seizure disorder.

REFERENCES

Back E, Voiculescu I, Brunger M, Wolff G. 1989. Familial ring (20) chromosomal mosaicism. *Hum. Genet.* 83:148–154.

Burnell RH, Stern LM, Sutherland G. 1985. A case of ring 20 chromosome with cardiac and renal anomalies. *Aust. Paediatr. J.* 21:285–286.

Borgaonkar DS, Lacassie YE, Stoll C. 1976. Usefullness of chromosome catalog in delineating new syndromes. Birth Defects Original Article Series XII (5): 87–95.

Callen DF, Eyre HJ, Ringenbergs ML, Freemantle CJ, Woodroffe P, Haan EA. 1991. Chromosomal origin of small ring marker chromosomes in man: characterization by molecular genetics. *Am. J. Hum. Genet.* 48:769–782.

Canevini MP, Sgro V, Zuffardi O, Canger R, Carrozzo R, Rossi E, Ledbetter D, Minicucci F, Vignoli A, Piazzini A, Guidolin L, Saltarelli A, dalla Bernardina B. 1998. Chromosome 20 ring: a chromosomal disorder associated with a particular electroclinical pattern. *Epilepsia.* 39:942–951.

Holopainen I, Penttinen M, Lakkala T, Aarimaa T. 1994. Ring chromosome 20 mosaicism in a girl with complex partial seizures. *Dev. Med. Child Neurol.* 36:70–73.

Inoue Y, Fujiwara T, Matsuda K, Kubota H, Tanaka M, Yagi K, Yamamori K, Takahashi Y. 1997. Ring chromosome 20 and nonconvulsive status epilepticus. A new epileptic syndrome. *Brain.* 120:939–953.

Kobayashi K, Inagaki M, Sasaki M, Sugai K, Ohta S, Hashimoto T. 1998. Characteristic EEG findings in ring 20 syndrome as a diagnostic clue. *Electroencephalogr. Clin. Neurophysiol.* 107:258–262.

Roubertie A, Petit J, Genton P. 2000. [Ring chromosome 20: an identifiable epileptic syndrome]. *Rev. Neurol.* 156:149–153.

CHROMOSOME 21 TRISOMY

Down Syndrome

Down syndrome, first described in 1866, is probably the most widely recognized malformation syndrome associated with mental retardation. It is the most common mental retardation syndrome recognizable at birth. Down syndrome occurs in about 1 in 700 newborns in most geographic regions, ethnic/racial groups, and all socioeconomic classes. Its chromosomal basis was recognized in 1959.

MAIN FEATURES: Infantile hypotonia, brachycephaly, upward slanting palpebral fissures, dysplastic ears, simian crease congenital heart defects, psychomotor retardation

GENERAL CHARACTERISTICS: The weight, length, and head size of birth are generally within the normal range. Generalized hypotonia is common in infants and newborns and may be associated with poor suck. Failure to thrive is more common when associated with cyanotic heart defect. Throughout childhood and adolescence height and head size tend to be in the lower percentiles with a tendency toward excessive weight for height.

ABNORMALITIES

Craniofacies: The facial features of Down syndrome are distinctive due to a round face, upward-slanted, small palpebral fissures, small, dysplastic auricles, short, upturned nose with depressed nasal bridge, and epicanthic folds. The mouth tends to be small. Newborns and infants manifest tongue-thrusting behavior, which is usually not due to a large tongue or small oral cavity. Brachycephaly, large fontanelle, delayed closure, and the presence of a third fontanelle in addition to the anterior and posterior are common. Dentition is remarkable for small, hypoplastic teeth with fewer caries but increased incidence of periodontal disease.

Brain: Gross anatomic malformations of the brain are remarkably uncommon in patients with trisomy 21 as compared to other chromosomal syndromes. However, impairment of overall congnitive ability is consistently present. There is a wide range of IQ noted throughout childhood with a mean of about 50. Adaptive and social skills are generally higher than verbal and mathematical abilities. Independent adult living with supervision is an achievable goal for a significant number of Down syndrome individuals. Behavior problems, attention-deficit hyperactivity disorder (ADHD), anxiety, depression, and seizures are not at all uncommon and require attention by specialists comfortable with managing these problems in mentally retarded individuals.

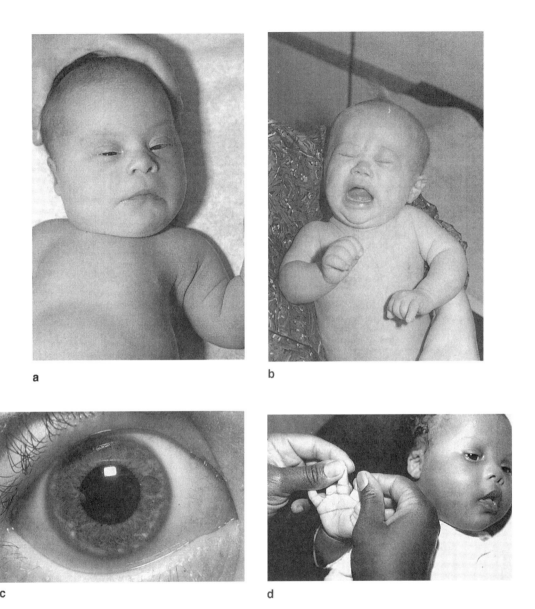

a   b

c   d

Newborn infant with Down syndrome. Note round head, round face, small upward-slanting palpebral fissures, downturned mouth, small chin (a), and crying facies, which is sometimes helpful in clinical diagnosis in mildly affected newborns (b). Brushfield spots, epicanthal fold (c), and transverse palmar crease, short, wide palm and fifth-finger clinodactyly (d) are additional features of diagnostic value.

Eyes: Brushfield spots, the speckled areas of hypoplastic peripheral iris, are noted in individuals with blue or light-colored irides and have no clinical morbidity associated with them. Refractive errors (myopia, astigmatism), strabismus, blockage of the lacrimal ducts, lenticular opacities, and cataracts are common enough that evaluation by an ophthalmologist during the first year of life is recommended for all infants with Down syndrome. Acquired cataracts at a young age are also common.

Limbs: Hands tend to be short and wide with shortened metacarpals and digits. Fifth-finger clinodactyly with a single flexion crease and a transverse palmar crease (simian crease) are of diagnostic value but cause no functional impairment. Increased space between the first and second toes is also common.

Heart: Heart defects, particularly involving the atrial and ventricular septa, occur in about 40–45% of newborns with Down syndrome. Echocardiographic evaluation of the heart should be carried out routinely in newborns and infants since heart defects are the major determinant of morbidity and mortality in infancy and childhood.

Organs: Gastrointestinal malformations including duodenal atresia, tracheoesophageal fistula, pyloric stenosis, annular pancreas, Hirschsprung disease, and imperforate anus occur in about 10–12% of the patients. Skeletal abnormalities such as hypoplasia of the odontoid process, incomplete fusion of spinal arches, hip dysplasia and 11 pairs of ribs are part of the Down syndrome phenotype.

Genitourinary: Hypoplasia of the penis and testicles and undescended testes may be present. Primary gonadal dysfunction associated with infertility is present in all males. Females with Down syndrome go through normal puberty and are fertile. Offspring of Down syndrome women have a high risk for aneuploidy. Both congenital and acquired hypothyroidism are more common than in the general population.

CYTOGENETICS: Full trisomy 21 resulting from maternal meiosis I nondisjunction is the most common cause of Down syndrome, accounting for about 95% of the cases. Mosaicism for trisomy 21 and normal cell lines is occasionally found (1–2%) but is not useful as a predictor of long-term prognosis. Robertsonian translocations involving a member of the D group (most commonly a 14) with a chromosome 21 may be found in about 5% of the cases. About 50% of these are inherited, more often from a balanced translocation carrier mother than the father. Other structural abnormalities such as G/G and non-Robertsonian translocations are rare. Genotype–phenotype correlation studies of partially trisomic individuals suggest that most of the common features of Down syndrome including congenital heart defects are attributable to band 21q22.3.

PRENATAL DIAGNOSIS: Down syndrome can be diagnosed prenatally by amniocentesis in early second trimester or by chorionic villus sampling in late first trimester. Noninvasive screening methods using maternal serum markers such as alpha-fetoprotein, chorionic gonadotropin and estriol, fetal sonography, maternal age and family history are used to identify pregnancies at high risk.

CLINICAL COURSE: The average life expectancy for Down syndrome in developed countries now exceeds 45 years. Early onset Alzheimer disease manifests by the fourth decade of life in a very high proportion of the patients. Atherosclerotic heart disease, alcohol and drug abuse may be less common than in the general population.

REFERENCES

American Academy of Pediatric Committee on Genetics. 1994. Health supervision for children with Down syndrome. American Academy of Pediatrics Committee on Genetics. *Pediatrics* 93:855–859.

Antonarakis SE. 1991. Parental origin of the extra chromosome in trisomy 21 as indicated by analysis of DNA polymorphisms. Down Syndrome Collaborative Group. *N. Engl. J. Med.* 324:872–876.

Baird PA, Sadovnick AD. 1987. Life expectancy in Down syndrome. *J. Pediatr.* 110:849–854.

Cooley WC, Graham JM Jr. 1991. Down syndrome—an update and review for the primary pediatrician. *Clin. Pediatr.* 30:233–253.

Cronk C, Crocker AC, Pueschel SM, Shea AM, Zackai E, Pickens G, Reed RB. 1988. Growth charts for children with Down syndrome: 1 month to 18 years of age. *Pediatrics.* 81:102–110.

Hennequin M, Allison PJ, Veyrune JL. 2000. Prevalence of oral health problems in a group of individuals with Down syndrome in France. *Dev. Med. Child Neurol.* 42:691–698.

Hook EB, Mutton DE, Ide R, Alberman E, Bobrow M. 1995. The natural history of Down syndrome conceptuses diagnosed prenatally that are not electively terminated. *Am. J. Hum. Genet.* 57:875–881.

Korenberg JR, Bradley C, Disteche CM. 1992. Down syndrome: molecular mapping of the congenital heart disease and duodenal stenosis. *Am. J. Hum. Genet.* 50:294–302.

Reeves RH, Baxter LL, Richtsmeier JT. 2001. Too much of a good thing: mechanisms of gene action in Down syndrome. *Trends Genet.* 17:83–88.

Rowley JD. 1981. Down syndrome and acute leukaemia: increased risk may be due to trisomy 21. *Lancet* 2:1020–1022.

Snijders RJ, Noble P, Sebire, N, Souka A, Nicolaides KH. 1998. UK multicentre project on assessment of risk of trisomy 21 by maternal age and fetal nuchal-translucency thickness at 10–14 weeks of gestation. Fetal Medicine Foundation First Trimester Screening Group. *Lancet* 352:343–346.

Wald NJ, Watt HC, Hackshaw AK. 1999. Integrated screening for Down's syndrome on the basis of tests performed during the first and second trimesters. *N. Engl. J. Med.* 341:461–467.

CHROMOSOME 21q COMPLETE MONOSOMY/PARTIAL MONOSOMY

With the exception of interstitial deletions involving only the juxta centromeric bands 21q11q21, complete or partial deletions of the long arm of chromosome 21 are associated with overlapping clinical manifestations that justify lumping them together. Partial monosomy 21q was first described by Lejeune et al. in 1964. Huret et al. (1995) provided a review of the phenotypic features of monosomy 21q based on 24 cases not associated with translocations or ring 21 chromosomes.

MAIN FEATURES: Mental retardation, growth retardation, microcephaly, large low-set ears

GENERAL CHARACTERISTICS: Most patients were born at term with only mild intrauterine growth retardation. Postnatal failure to thrive with growth between the third and tenth centile is common. Developmental delay associated with hypotonia or hypertonia is consistently present even though it varies from mild to severe in either partial or complete monosomy patients. An exceptional case with normal intelligence at 8 years old had an interstitial deletion of the 21q11.2q22.2 segment.

ABNORMALITIES

Craniofacies: Microcephaly, narrow, receding forehead, low hairline, prominent occiput are virtually constant. Narrow palpebral fissures with a downward slant, epicanthus, and hypertelorism are common. Microphthlamia is less common. Nose shows broad root, broad tip, absent furrow between alae nasi and the septum. Large, low-set ears with prominent antihelix and large lobule may be a distinctive feature of this syndrome. The mouth is large with long philtrum, thin vermillion, and highly arched or cleft palate in some cases. Microretrognathia is present in virtually all cases.

Limbs: Slender, overlapping fingers, arthrogryposis, and clubfoot are common. Simian creases have been reported but the data on dermatoglyphics are otherwise scarce.

Organs: Cardiac murmurs or anomalies and ambiguous genitalia have been found in 75% and 50% of the cases, respectively. Brain anomalies have included cerebral and cerebellar atrophy and thinning of the corpus callosum.

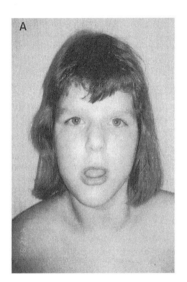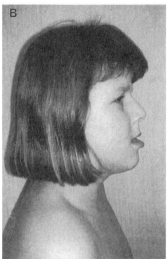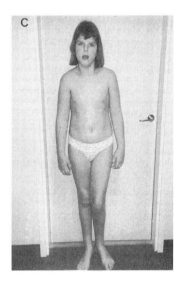

Girl at age 10 years and 6 months with proximal 21q monosomy involving bands 21q11.1q22.1. (From Ahlbom et al., 1966. *Am. J. Med. Genet.* 64:501–565. Copyright © 1966 John Wiley & Sons, Inc. Reprinted by permission of Wiley-Liss, Inc.)

CLINICAL COURSE: Patients with complete monosomy 21q died in infancy with only one patient reported to have lived until 11 years old. Patients with partial monosomy 21q fare better with survival to adulthood known in a few cases.

CYTOGENETICS: Monosomy 21q occurs most commonly in association with partial trisomy for another chromosome due to malsegregation of balanced translocations. De novo translocations also occur. When monosomy is due to a de novo deletion, the phenotype occurs in its purest form as described above.

Several cases of translocations involving 5p and distal 21q have been mistakenly identified as 21q partial monosomy. It has been suggested that awareness of this "5p/21q deletion" syndrome may minimize these diagnostic errors. Presence of the facial features of the cri-du-chat syndrome in patients with 21q partial monosomy may be a clue to suspect this syndrome.

REFERENCES

Ahlbom BE, Sidenvall R, Anneren G. 1996. Deletion of chromosome 21 in a girl with congenital hypothyroidism and mild mental retardation. *Am. J. Med. Genet.* 64:501–505.

Huret JL, Leonard C, Chery M, Philippe C, Schafei-Benaissa E, Lefaure G, Labrune B, Gilgenkrantz S. 1995. Monosomy 21q: two cases of del(21q) and review of the literature. *Clin. Genet.* 48:140–147.

Korenberg JR, Kalousek DK, Anneren G, Pulst SM, Hall JG, Epstein CJ, Cox DR. 1991. Deletion of chromosome 21 and normal intelligence: molecular definition of the lesion. *Hum. Genet.* 87:112–118.

Krasikov N, Takaesu N, Hassold T, Knops JF, Finley WH, Scarbrough P. 1992. Molecular and cytogenetic investigation of complex tissue-specific duplication and loss of chromosome 21 in a child with monosomy 21 phenotype. *Am. J. Med. Genet.* 43:554–560.

Phelan MC, Morton CC, Stevenson RE, Tanzi RE, Stewart GD, Watkins PC, Gusella JF, Amos JA. 1988. Molecular and cytogenetic characterization of a de novo t(5p;21q) in a patient previously diagnosed as monosomy 21. *Am. J. Hum. Genet.* 43:511–519.

Roland B, Cox DM, Hoar DI, Fowlow SB, Robertson AS. 1990. A familial interstitial deletion of the long arm of chromosome 21. *Clin. Genet.* 37:423–428.

Theodoropoulos DS, Cowan JM, Elias ER, Cole C. 1995. Physical findings in 21q22 deletion suggest critical region for 21q-phenotype in q22. *Am. J. Med. Genet.* 59:161–163.

Wisniewski K, Dambska M, Jenkins EC, Sklower S, Brown WT. 1983. Monosomy 21 syndrome: further delineation including clinical, neuropathological, cytogenetic and biochemical studies. *Clin. Genet.* 23:102–110.

RING CHROMOSOME 21

Ring chromosome 21 was first identified by Chandley in 1979 in a patient originally described by McIlree et al. in 1966. Like ring chromosomes associated with other autosomes the phenotypic features of ring 21 are highly variable and non-specific. Even though there is no unique clinical syndrome associated with ring 21, this not so uncommon karyotypic abnormality has important clinical consequences.

MAIN FEATURES: Developmental delay, flat nasal bridge, epicanthal folds, azoospermia

ABNORMALITIES

Craniofacial: Micrognathia, epicanthal folds, flat nasal bridge, low-set ears, everted lower lip

Limbs: Lymphedema of hands and feet, dysplastic toenails, normal dermatoglyphics

Central nervous system: Developmental delay, hypotonia, seizures

Genitourinary: Infertility, azoospermia

Other: Atrial septal defect, kyphosis

CLINICAL COURSE: Developmental delay has been variable and influenced by breakpoints and mosaicism. Clinically normal adults with r(21) chromosomes are known.

CYTOGENETICS: Most cases are sporadic. Familial cases are usually due to maternal transmission. Adult males with r(21) are usually infertile. Meiotic studies in a few cases have found failure of pairing at first meiotic division. Ring 21 chromosomes do not seem to affect female meiosis in the same manner. Transmission from phenotypically normal women heterozygous for ring 21 chromosomes with or without the presence of a normal cell line have been reported. Such women have a high risk for reproductive mishaps including offspring with ring 21 and trisomy 21. Duplications of segments within the ring may cause functional trisomy 21 and features of Down syndrome.

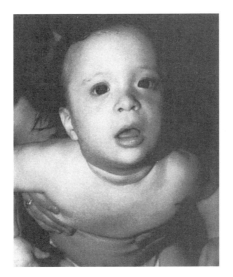

Patient with 45,XX,-21/46XX,-21,+ring(21) mosaicism and duplication of 21q21.1q22.2 within the ring, resulting in mild features of Down syndrome. (From Palmer et al., 1995. *Am. J. Med. Genet.* 57:527–536. Copyright © 1995 John Wiley & Sons, Inc. Reprinted by permission of Wiley-Liss, Inc.)

REFERENCES

Aronson DC, Jansweijer MC, Hoovers JM, Barth PG. 1987. A male infant with holoprosencephaly, associated with ring chromosome 21. *Clin. Genet.* 31:48–52.

Crusi A, Engel E. 1986. [Prenatal diagnosis of 3 cases of ring G chromosomes: one 21 and two 22, one of which was de novo]. *Ann. Genet.* 29:253–260.

Falik-Borenstein TC, Pribyl TM, Pulst SM, Van Dyke DL, Weiss L, Chu ML, Kraus J, Marshak D, Korenberg JR. 1992. Stable ring chromosome 21: molecular and clinical definition of the lesion. *Am. J. Med. Genet.* 42:22–28.

Kennerknecht I, Barbi G, Vogel W. 1990. Maternal transmission of ring chromosome 21. *Hum. Genet.* 86:99–101.

Kleczkowska A, Fryns JP. 1984. Ring chromosome 21 in a normal female. *Ann. Genet.* 27:126–128.

McGinniss MJ, Kazazian HH Jr, Stetten G, Petersen MB, Boman H, Engel E, Greenberg F, Hertz JM, Johnson A, Laca Z, et al. 1992. Mechanisms of ring chromosome formation in 11 cases of human ring chromosome 21. *Am. J. Hum. Genet.* 50:15–28.

Meire FM, Fryns JP. 1994. Lens dislocation and optic nerve hypoplasia in ring chromosome 21 mosaicism. *Ann. Genet.* 37:150–152.

Melnyk AR, Ahmed I, Taylor JC. 1995. Prenatal diagnosis of familial ring 21 chromosome. *Prenat. Diagn.* 15:269–273.

Miller K, Reimer A, Schulze B. 1987. Tandem duplication chromosome 21 in the offspring of a ring chromosome 21 carrier. *Ann. Genet.* 30:180–182.

Palmer CG, Blouin JL, Bull MJ, Breitfeld P, Vance GH, Van Meter T, Weaver DD, Heerema NA, Colbern SG, Korenberg JR, et al. 1995. Cytogenetic and molecular analysis of a ring (21) in a patient with partial trisomy 21 and megakaryocytic leukemia. *Am. J. Med. Genet.* 57:527–536.

Philip N, Baeteman MA, Mattei MG, Mattei JF. 1984. Three new cases of partial monosomy 21 resulting from one ring 21 chromosome and two unbalanced reciprocal translocations. *Eur. J. Pediatr.* 142:61–64.

CHROMOSOME 22 TRISOMY

Full trisomy 22 without mosaicism for a normal cell line is rarely found in live-born infants. The following summary is based on recent reviews by Bacino et al. (1995) and Crowe et al. (1997).

ABNORMALITIES

Craniofacies: Microcephaly, hypertelorism, epicanthal folds, and hypoplastic or low-set ears, ear pits, preauricular tags, cleft lip, and cleft palate

Limbs: Hypoplastic distal phalanges, digitalized thumbs, and clubfoot

Organs: Anal atresia or stenosis, cardiac, renal, and male genital anomalies, webbed neck with redundant skin, holoprosencephaly, and diaphragmatic hernia

CLINICAL COURSE:
All patients with full trisomy 22 died during infancy except for one who was 3 years old at the time of the report.

CYTOGENETICS:
All cases are sporadic. Mosaicism for a normal cell line is associated with longer survival.

REFERENCES

Bacino CA, Schreck R, Fischel-Ghodsian N, Pepkowitz S, Prezant TR, Graham JM Jr. 1995. Clinical and molecular studies in full trisomy 22: further delineation of the phenotype and review of the literature. *Am. J. Med. Genet.* 56:359–365.

Berghella V, Wapner RJ, Yang-Feng T, Mahoney MJ. 1998. Prenatal confirmation of true fetal trisomy 22 mosaicism by fetal skin biopsy following normal fetal blood sampling. *Prenat. Diagn.* 18:384–389.

Crowe CA, Schwartz S, Black CJ, Jaswaney V. 1997. Mosaic trisomy 22: a case presentation and literature review of trisomy 22 phenotypes. *Am. J. Med. Genet.* 71:406–413.

Fahmi F, Schmerler S, Hutcheon RG. 1994. Hydrocephalus in an infant with trisomy 22. *J. Med. Genet.* 31:141–144.

Feret MA, Galan F, Aguilar MS, Serrano JL, Cidras M, Garcia R. 1991. Full trisomy 22 in a malformed newborn female. *Ann. Genet.* 34:44–46.

Kobrynski L, Chitayat D, Zahed L, McGregor D, Rochon L, Brownstein S, Vekemans M, Albert DL. 1993. Trisomy 22 and facioauriculovertebral (Goldenhar) sequence. *Am. J. Med. Genet.* 46:68–71.

Kukolich MK, Kulharya A, Jalal SM, Drummond-Borg M. 1989. Trisomy 22: no longer an enigma. *Am. J. Med. Genet.* 34:541–544.

Ladonne JM, Gaillard D, Carre-Pigeon F, Gabriel R. 1996. Fryns syndrome phenotype and trisomy 22. *Am. J. Med. Genet.* 61:68–70.

Manasse BF, Pfaffenzeller WM, Gurtunca N, de Ravel TJ. 2000. Possible isochromosome 22 leading to trisomy 22. *Am. J. Med. Genet.* 95:411–414.

McPherson E, Stetka DG. 1990. Trisomy 22 in a liveborn infant with multiple congenital anomalies. *Am. J. Med. Genet.* 36:11–14.

Nicholl RM, Grimsley L, Butler L, Palmer RW, Rees HC, Savage MO, Costeloe K. 1994. Trisomy 22 and intersex. *Arch. Dis. Child Fetal Neonatal Ed.* 71:57–58.

Pridjian G, Gill WL, Shapira E. 1995. Goldenhar sequence and mosaic trisomy 22. *Am. J. Med. Genet.* 59:411–413.

Schinzel A. 1981. Incomplete trisomy 22. III. Mosaic-trisomy 22 and the propblem of full trisomy 22. *Hum. Genet.* 56:269–273.

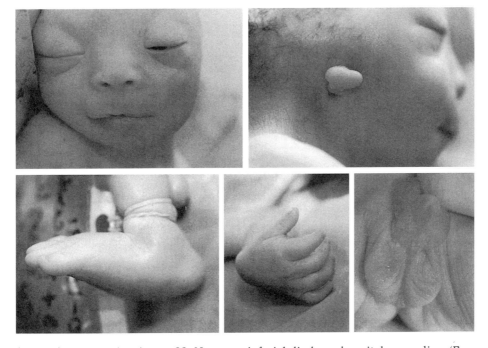

An infant with nonmosaic trisomy 22. Note craniofacial, limb, and genital anomalies. (From Bacino et al., 1995. *Am. J. Med. Genet.* 56:359–365. Copyright © 1995 John Wiley & Sons, Inc. Reprinted by permission of Wiley-Liss, Inc.)

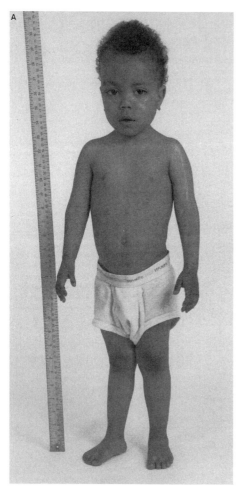
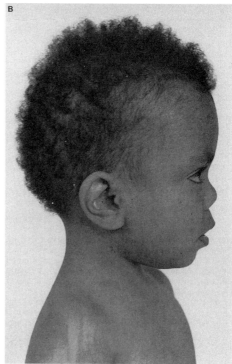

Boy at 4 years and 9 months with trisomy 22 mosaicism and a minimally abnormal phenotype was identified because of developmental delay, growth failure, mild facial and limb anomalies, and whirling hypopigmentation. Peripheral blood and skin fibroblasts showed 4% and 90%+ cells with trisomy 22, respectively. (From Crowe et al., 1997. *Am. J. Med. Genet.* 71:406–413. Copyright © 1997 John Wiley & Sons, Inc. Reprinted by permission of Wiley-Liss, Inc.)

CHROMOSOME 22pTER → q11 TRISOMY/TETRASOMY

Cat-Eye Syndrome

The multiple malformation syndrome consisting of coloboma of the iris, preauricular tags and pits, anal atresia, congenital cardiac and renal malformations, and a supernumerary marker chromosome derived from chromosome 22 has been designated the Cat-Eye syndrome. A single malformation that is not always present, that is, the iris coloboma, is overemphasized by this designation.

MAIN FEATURES: Iris coloboma, ear anomalies, anorectal anomalies, congenital heart defects.

ABNORMALITIES

Craniofacies: Coloboma of the iris, choroid, and retina, downward-slanting palpebral fissures, microphthalmia, preauricular skin tags or sinuses, and small pinnae

Organs: Congenital heart defects, particularly total anomalous pulmonary venous return (TAPVR)—a rare form of congenital heart defect—is common in this syndrome. Renal malformation or absence of a kidney may be seen. Anal atresia with or without fistula is one of the original defining characteristics of the syndrome.

Other: Growth is usually normal. Developmental delay and mental retardation can vary from mild to severe. Normal intelligence has also been reported.

CYTOGENETICS: Effective trisomy or tetrasomy for the 22pter → q11.2 segment usually due to the presence of a supernumerary submetacentric or metacentric, bisatellited chromosome. Inverted duplication of 22pter → q11 region appears to be the most common mechanism. Interstitial duplication of 22q11.2q12 and 22q11.1q11.2 have been reported. A minute supernumerary double ring derived from 22q11.2 has also caused a similar clinical phenotype in at least one patient and variable manifestations in his family.

Molecular studies have marked the distal boundary of the Cat-Eye syndrome to 22q11.2 proximal to the DiGeorge syndrome (DGS) locus. Triplication as well as quadruplication of 22q11 loci has been documented. A dosage effect may correlate with the severity of the clinical phenotype. Mosaicism also impacts on the expression of the phenotype.

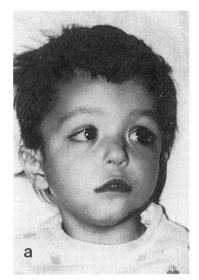
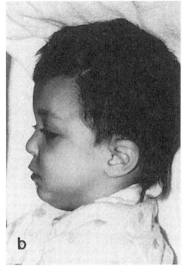

Downward-slanted palpebral fissures, epicanthal folds, low-set ears, and preauricular pits are seen in this boy with interstitial duplication of 22q11. He also had TAPVR, scrotal anomalies, and an absent kidney. (From Knoll et al., 1995. *Am. J. Med. Genet.* 55:221–224. Copyright © 1995 John Wiley & Sons, Inc. Reprinted by permission of Wiley-Liss, Inc.)

REFERENCES

Cullen P, Rodgers CS, Callen DF, Connolly VM, Eyre H, Fells P, Gordon H, Winter RM, Thakker RV. 1993. Association of familial Duane anomaly and urogenital abnormalities with a bisatellited marker derived from chromosome 22. *Am. J. Med. Genet.* 47:925–930.

Knoll JH, Asamoah A, Pletcher BA, Wagstaff J. 1995. Interstitial duplication of proximal 22q: phenotypic overlap with cat eye syndrome. *Am. J. Med. Genet.* 55:221–224.

Magenis RE, Sheehy RR, Brown MG, McDermid HE, White BN, Zonana J, Weleber R. 1988. Parental origin of the extra chromosome in the cat eye syndrome: evidence from heteromorphism and in situ hybridization analysis. *Am. J. Med. Genet.* 29:9–19.

Mears AJ, Duncan AM, Budarf ML, Emanuel BS, Sellinger S, Siegel-Bartelt J, Greenberg CR, McDermid HE. 1994. Molecular characterization of the marker chromosome associated with cat eye syndrome. *Am. J. Hum. Genet.* 55:134–142.

Reiss JA, Weleber RG, Brown MG, Bangs CD, Lovrien EW, Magenis RE. 1985. Tandem duplication of proximal 22q: a cause of cat-eye syndrome. *Am. J. Med. Genet.* 20:165–171.

Schinzel A, Schmid W, Fraccaro M, Tiepolo L, Zuffardi O, Opitz JM, Lindsten J, Zetterqvist P, Enell H, Baccichetti C, Tenconi R, Pagon RA. 1981. The "cat eye syndrome": dicentric small marker chromosome probably derived from a no. 22 (tetrasomy 22pter to q11) associated with a characteristic phenotype. Report of 11 patients and delineation of the clinical picture. *Hum. Genet.* 57:148–158.

Wenger SL, Surti U, Nwokoro NA, Steele MW. 1994. Cytogenetic characterization of cat eye syndrome marker chromosome. *Ann. Genet.* 37:33–36.

CHROMOSOME 22q PROXIMAL MONOSOMY

Deletion within chromosome band 22q11 is probably among the most common chromosomal abnormalities associated with a recognizable pattern of malformation. The estimated incidence is about 1:5000 births and 1:20 cases of congenital heart defects.

Many clinically defined syndromes, including the DiGeorge syndrome, velocardiofacial syndrome, conotruncal facies syndrome, Cayler syndrome, and Opitz G/BBB syndrome, are associated with 22q11 deletion.

MAIN FEATURES: Conotruncal heart defects, facial anomalies, small ears, cleft palate, thymic hypoplasia

GENERAL CHARACTERISTICS: Newborns and infants may be recognized by the presence of any of the major anomalies represented by the acronym CATCH for cardiac abnormality, abnormal facies, thymic hypoplasia, cleft palate, and hypocalcemia. Older children and adults are identified when facial features associated with the velocardiofacial syndrome, bifid uvula, submucous cleft, velopharyngeal insufficiency, developmental or behavioral problems are investigated.

ABNORMALITIES:

Craniofacies: Hypertelorism, small ears, small mouth, round, small chin, and rounded cheeks with persistent buccal pads are common in infants. In older children and particularly in adults, maxillary and or mandibular prognathism and a long, tubular nose with bulbous tip are more common. There is a high degree of intrafamily and interfamilial variability in clinical expression. It has been suggested that there may be greater difficulty in recognition of the syndrome in African Americans.

Organs: Cardiac defects are found in about 70–75% of the patients. Tetralogy of Fallot, interrupted aortic arch, and other conotruncal anomalies and septal defects account for >90% of the cardiac defects. Hypoplastic left heart and double-outlet right ventricle are rarely seen. Cleft palate, bifid uvula, submucous cleft, and renal anomalies occur in 30% to 70% of the patients. A variety of other malformations, major and minor, have been associated with the 22q11 deletion syndrome.

Other: Hypocalcemia when present is usually found in infants, resolves by 3–4 years of age, and only rarely recurs. A deficiency of thymus-derived lymphocytes

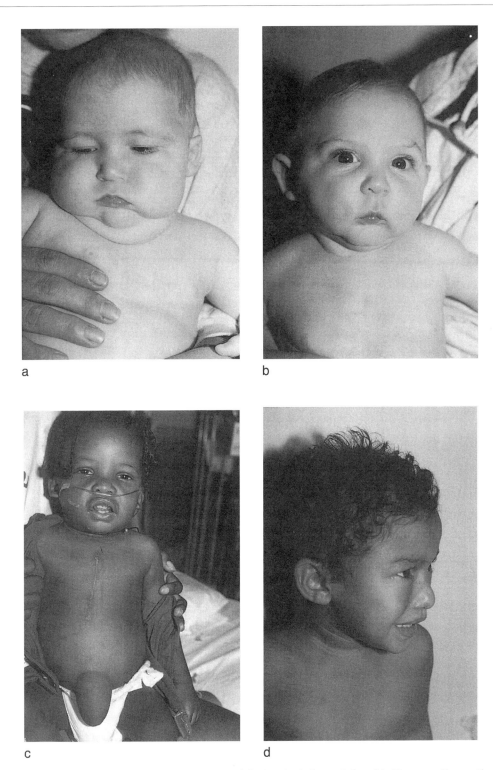

a   b

c   d

Facial features associated with 22q11.2 microdeletion in infants (a,b,c,d,). Note small mouth, small chin, prominent nasal bridge, widely spaced eyes, and minimally malformed ears.

(T cells) is present in 50–60% of the patients. B-cell deficiency may also be present. Serious infections, however, are not as common as might be expected on the basis of those laboratory abnormalities. A polyarthritis mimicking juvenile rheumatoid arthritis appears to be common in 22q11 deletion patients.

Brain: Learning disability, particularly in nonverbal communication, is present in a high proportion of children. IQ tests reveal most patients to be performing in the low normal, borderline, or mild range of retardation. Psychotic illnesses including schizophrenia, bipolar disorder, and depression appear to be more prevalent in adolescents and adults with this syndrome.

CYTOGENETICS: Most cases are due to submicroscopic deletions detectable by fluorescence in situ hybridization (FISH) using a DiGeorge syndrome critical region (DGCR) probe. High-resolution cytogenetics may reveal visible deletions but this test is not sensitive enough for diagnostic purposes. Most cases arise de novo. About 6–10% of the cases are familial. Since there is great variability in the phenotypic expression of this syndrome, clinical assessments alone should not be relied on to detect familial cases. FISH studies of parents and other relatives of index cases are recommended. There is a low but unquantified risk of germline mosaicism and recurrence of 22q11 for parents who have normal FISH test results. Offspring of affected patients have 50% risk of inheriting the deletion.

REFERENCES

Driscoll DA, Budarf ML, Emanuel BS. 1992. A genetic etiology for DiGeorge syndrome: consistent deletions and microdeletions of 22q11. *Am. J. Hum. Genet.* 50:924–933.

McDonald-McGinn DM, Kirschner R, Goldmuntz E, Sullivan K, Eicher P, Gerdes M, Moss E, Solot C, Wang P, Jacobs I, Handler S, Knightly C, Heher K, Wilson M, Ming JE, Grace K, Driscoll D, Pasquariello P, Randall P, Larossa D, Emanuel BS, Zackai EH. 1999. The Philadelphia story: the 22q11.2 deletion: report on 250 patients. *Genet. Couns.* 10:11–24.

Sullivan KE, McDonald-McGinn DM, Driscoll DA, Zmijewski CM, Ellabban AS, Reed L, Emanuel BS, Zackai EH, Athreya BH, Keenan G. 1997. Juvenile rheumatoid arthritis-like polyarthritis in chromosome 22q11.2 deletion syndrome (DiGeorge anomalad/velocardiofacial syndrome/conotruncal anomaly face syndrome). *Arthritis Rheum.* 40:430–436.

Wang PP, Solot C, Moss EM, Gerdes M, McDonald-McGinn DM, Driscoll DA, Emanuel BS, Zackai EH. 1998. Developmental presentation of 22q11.2 deletion (DiGeorge/velocardiofacial syndrome). *J. Dev. Behav. Pediatr.* 19:342–345.

Wilson DI, Burn J, Scambler P, Goodship J. 1993. DiGeorge syndrome: part of CATCH 22. *J. Med. Genet.* 30:852–856.

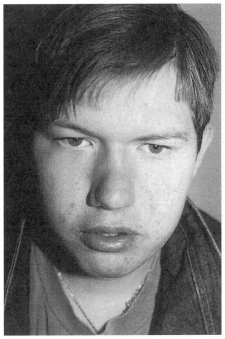
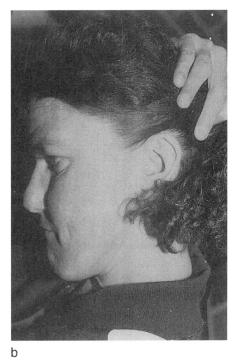

a   b

A teenager (a) and his mother (b), both with 22q11.2 microdeletion. Note characteristic tubular nose, maxillary prognathism, and normal ears.

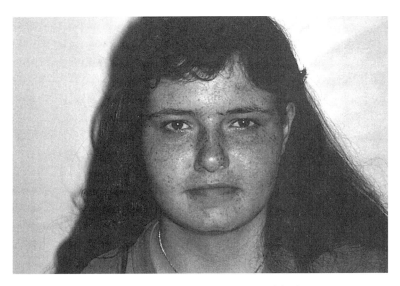

Note the remarkable variability of this syndrome. This normal-looking young woman was identified as having submucous cleft palate and 22q11.2 microdeletion after she had a baby with tetralogy of Fallot.

CHROMOSOME 22q DISTAL MONOSOMY
22q13 Deletion Syndrome

Partial deletions of the long arm of chromosome 22 appear to be relatively common. At least two distinct clinical entities, the 22q11 deletion syndrome and the 22q13 deletion syndrome, are recognizable. This summary is based on 61 cases of 22q13 deletions studied and reviewed by Phelan et al. (2001).

MAIN FEATURES: Severe psychomotor retardation, normal or accelerated growth, dolichocephaly, dysplastic ears

GENERAL CHARACTERISTICS: Severe to profound mental retardation and absent or severely delayed speech is present in >90% of the cases. Growth is described as normal or accelerated in about 88% of the cases.

ABNORMALITIES

Craniofacies: Dolichocephaly (50%), prominent dysplastic ears (60%), ptosis (40%), epicanthal folds (40%), and a pointed chin (48%) are the most common findings. Cleft lip and cleft palate do not appear to be associated with 22q13 deletion.

Limbs: Hypoplastic toe nails (75%), large, fleshy hands (60%), syndactyly of second and third toes, and clinodactyly of the fifth fingers are the most common findings.

Other: Generalized hypotonia, increased tolerance to pain, chewing on clothes, toys, and other objects, and autistic behavior are frequently noted.

CLINICAL COURSE: Survival to adulthood known.

CYTOGENETICS: About 75% of the cases are due to simple terminal deletions of the band 22q13 and the remainder have been secondary to unbalanced translocations, de novo as well as familial, interstitial deletion and recombination within inversion 22 in a parent. There has been no phenotypic difference noted between maternally and paternally transmitted cases. A noteworthy feature is the high proportion of cases that are missed on initial studies of peripheral lymphocytes and amniocytes.

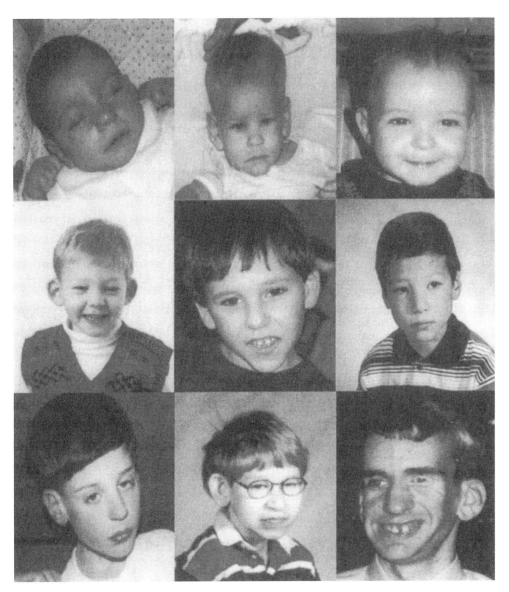

Facial appearance of 22q13 deletion patients from infancy to adulthood. (From Phelan et al., 2001. *Am. J. Med. Genet.* 22:283–287. Copyright © 2001 John Wiley & Sons, Inc. Reprinted by permission of Wiley-Liss, Inc.)

REFERENCES

Doheny KF, McDermid HE, Harum K, Thomas GH, Raymond GV. 1997. Cryptic terminal rearrangement of chromosome 22q13.32 detected by FISH in two unrelated patients. *J. Med. Genet.* 34:640–644.

Nesslinger NJ, Gorski JL, Kurczynski TW, Shapira SK, Cullen RF Jr, French BN, McDermid HE. 1994. Clinical, cytogenetic, and molecular characterization of seven patients with deletions of chromosome 22q13.3. *Am. J. Hum.* 54:464–472.

Phelan MC, Rogers RC, Saul RA, Stapleton GA, Sweet K, McDermid H, Shaw SR, Claytor J, Willis J, Kelly DP. 2001. 22q13 deletion syndrome. *Am. J. Med. Genet.* 101:91–99.

Watt JL, Olson IA, Johnston AW, Ross HS, Couzin DA, Stephen GS. 1985. A familial pericentric inversion of chromosome 22 with a recombinant subject illustrating a 'pure' partial monosomy syndrome. *J. Med. Genet.* 22:283–287.

RING CHROMOSOME 22

MAIN FEATURES: Psychomotor retardation, microcephaly, poor growth, absence of major malformation

GENERAL CHARACTERISTICS: Ring chromosome 22 is usually identified in patients studies for developmental delay. Poor growth is common. A characteristic dysmorphologic syndrome has not been established.

ABNORMALITIES

Craniofacial: Mild microcephaly, synophrys, epicanthal folds, long eyelashes, large ears, dental malocclusion

Limbs: Short, wide hands, syndactyly, brachydactyly, clinodactyly of the fifth fingers

Central nervous system: Microcephaly, hypotonia, moderate to profound mental retardation, ataxia, unsteady gait, and seizures

Other: Constitutional ring chromosome 22 has been found in patients with meningioma, neurofibromatosis type II, metachromatic leukodystrophy, Cat-Eye syndrome and DiGeorge syndrome. Ring 22 and monosomy 22 are known to be acquired abnormalities in meningiomas.

CLINICAL COURSE: Survival to adulthood is common.

CYTOGENETICS: Most cases are sporadic. Familial transmission has occurred.

REFERENCES

Coulter-Mackie MB, Rip J, Ludman MD, Beis J, Cole DE. 1995. Metachromatic leucodystrophy (MLD) in a patient with a constitutional ring chromosome 22. *J. Med. Genet.* 32:787–791.

Frizzley JK, Stephan MJ, Lamb AN, Jonas PP, Hinson RM, Moffitt DR, Shkolny DL, McDermid HE. 1999. Ring 22 duplication/deletion mosaicism: clinical, cytogenetic, and molecular characterisation. *J. Med. Genet.* 36:237–241.

MacLean JE, Teshima IE, Szatmari P, Nowaczyk MJ. 2000. Ring chromosome 22 and autism: report and review. *Am. J. Med. Genet.* 90:382–385.

Mears AJ, el-Shanti H, Murray JC, McDermid HE, Patil SR. 1995. Minute supernumerary ring chromosome 22 associated with cat eye syndrome: further delineation of the critical region. *Am. J. Hum. Genet.* 57:667–673.

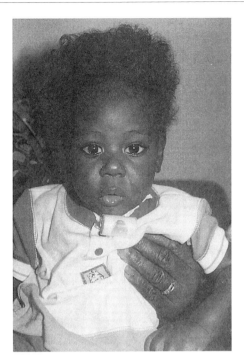

Infant with ring (22)/monosomy 22. Low birth weight, failure to thrive, small eyes, high nasal bridge, large, low-set ears, and profound global developmental delay were the clinical findings noted in this child.

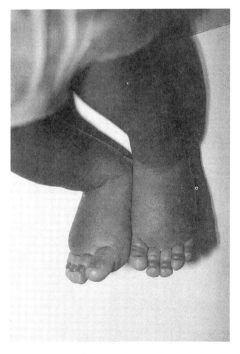

Infant with ring (22)/monosomy 22. Showing puffy feet due to dorsal lymphedema.

Petrella R, Levine S, Wilmot PL, Ashar KD, Casamassima AC, Shapiro LR. 1993. Multiple meningiomas in a patient with constitutional ring chromosome 22. *Am. J. Med. Genet.* 47:184–186.

Stoll C, Roth MP. 1983. Segregation of a 22 ring chromosome in three generations. *Hum. Genet.* 63:294–296.

Wenger SL, Boone LY, Cummins JH, Del Vecchio MA, Bay CA, Hummel M, Mowery-Rushton PA. 2000. Newborn infant with inherited ring and de novo interstitial deletion on homologous chromosome 22s. *Am. J. Med. Genet.* 91:351–354.

CHROMOSOME 47,XXY AND 48,XXYY SYNDROME

Klinefelter Syndrome

Originally described in 1942 by Klinefelter et al., this syndrome has an estimated incidence of about 1:500 male births. Even though hypogonadism and infertility are the primary clinical manifestations, additional somatic findings may be present as well.

GENERAL CHARACTERISTICS: Males with 47,XXY appear normal at birth and usually are not recognized until adolescence or young adulthood. Their height tends to be above average due to long limbs. Radioulnar synostosis and fifth-finger clinodactyly may be present. Taurodontism, crowns of permanent teeth larger than controls, has been documented. Children and adolescents may need counseling for poor school performance or behavioral problems.

ABNORMALITIES

Central nervous system: Mental retardation is not a part of the 47,XXY syndrome. However, full-scale and performance IQs tend to be below average, especially in relation to siblings with normal karyotypes. Children and adolescents with 47,XXY are more likely to be described as immature, shy, insecure, and having poor judgment. Patients with 48,XXYY or 48,XXXY karyotypes show greater cognitive dysfunction. Radio-ulnar synostosis is common in those patients.

Genitourinary: Primary hypogonadism due to atrophic testes and high levels of gonadotropins are usually present. Gynecomastia occurs in about 30% of adolescents with this syndrome. Gynecoid habitus may be present. Secondary sexual characteristics may be underdeveloped. Azoospermia is constant in the nonmosaic 47,XXY male. Precocious puberty and failure of puberty are common. Testosterone therapy may be needed in adolescents and young adults to induce and maintain masculinization and libido.

CLINICAL COURSE: Adults with 47,XXY Klinefelter syndrome are at increased risk for diabetes mellitus, obesity, carcinoma of the breast, germ cell tumors, and hypostatic leg ulceration.

CYTOGENETICS: The extra X chromosome in Klinefelter syndrome males is of maternal origin in about two-thirds of the cases and paternal in the rest. There is no parent-of-origin effect known. Maternal age may be a factor in the nondisjunctional error. Paternal age effect has not been found.

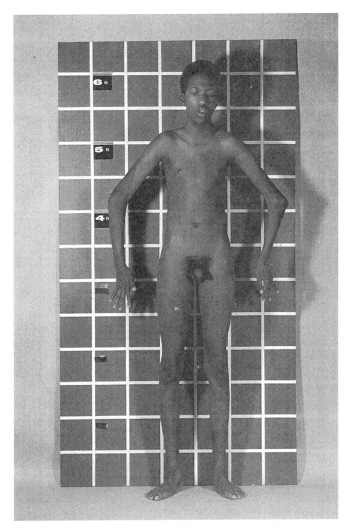

Boy 14 years of age with Klinefelter syndrome variant showing tall stature, long limbs, and contractures of elbows associated with 48,XXYY karyotype.

REFERENCES

Alvesalo L, Portin P. 1980. 47,XXY males: sex chromosomes and tooth size. *Am. J. Hum. Genet.* 32:955–959.

Bertelloni S, Baroncelli GI, Battini R, Saggese G. 1996. Central precocious puberty in Klinefelter syndrome: a case report with longitudinal follow-up of growth pattern. *Am. J. Med. Genet.* 65:52–55.

Borgaonkar DS, Mules EH, Char F. 1970. Do the 48,XXYY males have a characteristic phenotype? A review. *Clin. Genet.* 1:272–293.

Caldwell PD, Smith DW. 1972. The XXY (Klinefelter's) syndrome in childhood: detection and treatment. *J. Pediatr.* 80:250–258.

Campbell WA, Newton MS, Price WH. 1980. Hypostatic leg ulceration and Klinefelter's syndrome. *J. Ment. Defic. Res.* 24:115–117.

Ferguson-Smith M, Johnston AW, Handmaker SD. 1960. Primary amentia and micro-orchidism associated with an XXXY sex-chromosome constitution. Lancet II: 126–128.

Klinefelter HF Jr., Refenstein EC Jr. Albright F. 1942. Syndrome characterized by gynecomastia, spermatogenetic without aleydigism and increased excretion of follicle-stimulating hormone. *J. Clin. Endocrinol.* 2:615–627.

Robinson A, Lubs HA, Nielsen J, Sorensen. 1979. Summary of clinical findings: profiles of children with 47,XXY, 47,XXX and 47,XYY karyotypes. *Birth Defects* 15:261–266.

Salbenblatt JA, Meyers DC, Bender BG, Linden MG, Robinson A. 1987. Gross and fine motor development in 47,XXY and 47,XYY males. *Pediatrics* 80:240–244.

CHROMOSOME 49,XXXXX SYNDROME
Penta X Syndrome

First reported by Kesaree and Wooley (1963), the Penta X syndrome appears to be rarer than its male counterpart—the 49,XXXXY syndrome—judging by the number of reported cases.

MAIN FEATURES: Developmental delay, short stature, upward-slanting palpebral fissures, epicanthal folds, dysplastic ears.

GENERAL CHARACTERISTICS: Prenatal and postnatal growth deficiency is common, particularly affecting length.

ABNORMALITIES

Central nervous system: Mental retardation is always present. The severity varies. Measured IQs have ranged from 20 to 75.

Craniofacies: Microcephaly, upward-slanting palpebral fissures, low, broad nasal bridge, epicanthal folds, hypertelorism and dysplastic ears are commonly found, which is similar to the 49,XXXXY syndrome. Dental anomalies including taurodontism and enamel defects are also commonly found.

Genitourinary: Unlike their male counterparts, the 49,XXXXX females show no abnormality of external genitalia. Small uterus, ovarian dysfunction, and urinary tract abnormality are common.

Limbs: Small hands and feet, overlapping toes, clinodactyly of the fifth fingers, radioulnar synostosis, and ear joints are seen in about 50% of the patients. Talipes equino-varus, metatarsus varus, and scoliosis are less frequent.

Organs: Congenital heart defects, mostly patent ductus arteriosus (PDA) and septal defects, were found in 13 out of 23 cases reviewed by Cassia et al. (1991)

CYTOGENETICS: Maternal meiotic nondisjunction is responsible for the extra X chromosomes in all cases studied. One mother of a Penta X female had 47,XXX in 1 out of 50 examined cells. No mosaicism or other evidence of a tendency toward nondisjunction has been found. Maternal age effect has not been reported.

REFERENCES

Deng HX, Abe K, Kondo I, Tsukahara M, Inagaki H, Hamada I, Fukushima Y, Niikawa N. 1991. Parental origin and mechanism of formation of polysomy X: an XXXXX case and four XXXXY cases determined with RFLPs. *Hum. Genet.* 86:541–544.

Dryer RF, Patil SR, Zellweger HU, Simpson JM, Hanson JW, Aschenbrenner C, Weinstein SL. 1979. Pentasomy X with multiple dislocations. *Am. J. Med. Genet.* 4:313–321.

Fragoso R, Hernandez A, Plascencia ML, Nazara Z, Martinez y Martinez R, Cantu JM. 1982. 49,XXXXX syndrome. *Ann. Genet.* 25:145–148.

Funderburk SJ, Valente M, Klisak I. 1981. Pentasomy X: report of patient and studies of X-inactivation. *Am. J. Med. Genet.* 8:27–33.

Kasaree N, Wooley PV. 1963. A phenotypic female with 49 chromosomes, presumably XXXXX. A case report. *J. Pediatr.* 63:1099–1103.

Kassai R, Hamada I, Furuta H, Cho K, Abe K, Deng HX, Niikawa N. 1991. Penta X syndrome: a case report with review of the literature. *Am. J. Med. Genet.* 40:51–56.

Leal CA, Belmont JW, Nachtman R, Cantu JM, Medina C. 1994. Parental origin of the extra chromosomes in polysomy X. *Hum. Genet.* 94:423–426.

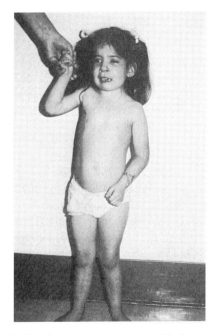

Five-year-old female with markedly short stature, ptosis of left upper eyelid, and genu valgus. She was microcephalic and developmentally delayed. (From Funderbunk et al., 1981. *Am. J. Med. Genet.* 8:27–33. Copyright © 1981 John Wiley & Sons, Inc. Reprinted by permission of Wiley-Liss, Inc.)

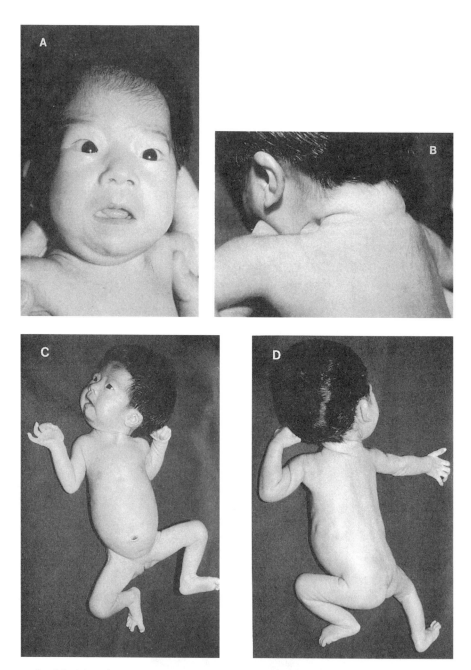

Four-month-old girl with microcephaly, narrow forehead, hirsutism, depressed, broad nasal bridge, upward-slanted palpebral fissures, redundant nuchal skin, low hairline, fifth-finger clinodactyly, and increased space between first and second toes. (From Kassai et al., 1991. *Am. J. Med. Genet.* 40:51–56. Copyright © 1991 John Wiley & Sons, Inc. Reprinted by permission of Wiley-Liss, Inc.)

Linden MG, Bender BG, Robinson A. 1995. Sex chromosome tetrasomy and pentasomy. *Pediatrics* 96:672–682.

Martini G, Carillo G, Catizone F, Notarangelo A, Mingarelli R, Dallapiccola B. 1993. On the parental origin of the X's in a prenatally diagnosed 49,XXXXX syndrome. *Prenat. Diagn.* 13:763–766.

Monheit A, Francke U, Saunders B, Jones KL. 1980. The penta-X syndrome. *J. Med. Genet.* 17:392–396.

Toussi T, Halal F, Lesage R, Delorme F, Bergeron A. 1980. Brief clinical report: renal hypodysplasia and unilateral ovarian agenesis in the penta-X syndrome. *Am. J. Med. Genet.* 6:153–162.

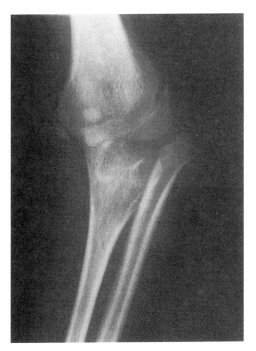 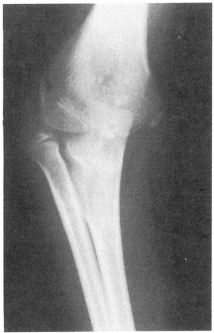

Ten-year-old girl with dislocation of the radial head and fusion of the proximal radius and ulna is shown in this radiograph. (From Dryer et al., 1979. *Am. J. Med. Genet.* 4:313–321. Copyright © 1979 John Wiley & Sons, Inc. Reprinted by permission of Wiley-Liss, Inc.)

CHROMOSOME 49,XXXXY SYNDROME

This relatively rare multiple X and single Y sex chromosome aneuploidy should not be considered a Klinefelter variant because the phenotype is quite distinctive. Both physical abnormalities and cognitive dysfunctions are much more severe than those found in the typical patients with 47,XXY karyotypes. The 48,XXXY may be more akin to the Klinefelter syndrome in this regard. This summary is based on more than 100 published cases. First described by Fraccaro et al. (1960), the 49,XXXXY syndrome has an estimated incidence of 1 in 85,000 live births.

MAIN FEATURES: Psychomotor retardation, upward slanting palpebral fissures, epicanthal folds, genital hypoplasia

ABNORMALITIES

Craniofacies: Widely spaced eyes, upward-slanted palpebral fissures, epicanthal folds, low nasal bridge, small nose with anteverted nares, and dysplastic ears are reported in 50% or more of the patients. Even though many of these features may be seen in Down syndrome, the overall appearance is quite dissimilar to Down syndrome. Cleft lip and palate also occur.

Limbs: Radioulnar synostosis associated with several sex chromosome aneuploidies is common in this syndrome as well. Fifth-finger clinodactyly, hypoplastic phalanges, hip dysplasia, coxa valga, genu valgus, and flat feet are frequently found. Mild epiphyseal dysplasia and delayed ossification of the bones may be found. Low total fingertip dermal ridge count is a consistent finding. Abnormal overlapping toes have also been noted.

Genitourinary: Hypoplastic scrotum, small penis, scrotalization of the penis, and cryptorchidism are present in 20–80% of the cases.

Central nervous system: Mental retardation is usually present but has varied in severity with measured IQ reported in the mild to profoundly retarded range. A striking discrepancy between expressive and receptive language development has been reported. Longitudinal studies have found deterioration of cognitive function by adulthood.

Organs: Congenital heart defects are present in about 18% of the cases, patent ductus being the most common. Septal defects, tetralogy of Fallot, and mitral valve prolapse have also been reported.

Other: Arhinencephaly, hypoplasia of the corpus callosum, hypoplastic inverted nipples, pectus excavatum, umbilical hernia, scoliosis

CYTOGENETICS: The origin of the extra X chromosomes has been traced to successive nondisjunction in maternal meiosis I and II in a few cases studied by molecular methods. No instances of maternal mosaicism for X-aneuploidy have been reported.

REFERENCES

Curfs LM, Schreppers-Tijdink G, Wiegers A, Borghgraef M, Fryns JP. 1990. The 49,XXXXY syndrome: clinical and psychological findings in five patients. *J. Ment. Defic. Res.* 34:277–282.

Fraccaro M, Kaisjer K, Lindsten J. 1966. A child with 49 chromosomes. *Lancet* II:899–902.

Huang TH, Greenberg F, Ledbetter DH. 1991. Determination of the origin of nondisjunction in a 49,XXXXY male using hypervariable dinucleotide repeat sequences. *Hum. Genet.* 86:619–620.

Karsh RB. 1975. Congenital heart disease in 49,XXXXY syndrome. *Pediatrics* 56:462–464.

Kleczkowska A, Fryns JP, Van den Berghe H. 1988. X-chromosome polysomy in the male. The Leuven experience 1966–1987. *Hum. Genet.* 80:16–22.

Leal CA, Belmont JW, Nachtman R, Cantu JM, Medina C. 1994. Parental origin of the extra chromosomes in polysomy X. *Hum. Genet.* 94:423–426.

Lomelino CA, Reiss A. 1991. 49,XXXXY syndrome: behavioural and developmental profiles. *J. Med. Genet.* 28:609–612.

Peet J, Weaver DD, Vance GH. 1998. 49,XXXXY: a distinct phenotype. Three new cases and review. *J. Med. Genet.* 35:420–424.

Sarto GE, Otto PG, Kuhn EM, Therman E. 1987. What causes the abnormal phenotype in a 49,XXXXY male? *Hum. Genet.* 75:1–4.

Sijmons RH, van Essen AJ, Visser JD, Iprenburg M, Nelck GF, Vos-Bender ML, de Jong B. 1995. Congenital knee dislocation in a 49,XXXXY boy. *J. Med. Genet.* 32:309–311.

CHROMOSOME 47,XYY AND 48,XYYY SYNDROME

Multiple Y Syndrome

The presence of a Y chromosome generally leads to male differentiation regardless of the number of X chromosomes present in humans. Chromosome 47,XYY is a common aneuploidy occurring in about 1:1000 male live births but rarely diagnosed in clinical settings due to its mild and nonspecific phenotypic effects.

48,XYYY is much rarer than 47,XYY. Its incidence is not known. These males have been identified by chromosomal studies performed because of radioulnar synostosis, lack of sexual desire, infertility, azoospermia, mild cognitive impairment, or mental illness.

Their physical appearance is characterized by tall stature, long face, large ears, epicanthal folds, flat nasal bridge, full lower lip, long philtrum, high palate, and short neck. Café-au-lait spots have been reported. Testicular atrophy was associated with lack of sexual desire in one 29-year-old male with 48,XYYY.

MAIN FEATURES: Above average height, absence of malformation and psychomotor retardation

GENERAL CHARACTERISTICS: Birth weight and length are generally normal with slight acceleration of linear growth noted between 4 and 6 years of age. On average, adult males with 47,XYY are taller than 46,XY males.

ABNORMALITIES

Craniofacies: Craniofacial features are not particularly abnormal. Prominent glabella, larger than normal tooth size, and large pinnae may be present.

Limbs: There are no characteristic dermatoglyphic or other abnormalities associated with this aneuploidy. However, radioulnar synostosis and restricted supination of the elbows may be seen as in other aneuploidies involving the X or the Y chromosome.

Other: No central nervous system (CNS) malformations occur as a part of this syndrome. However, EEG abnormalities have been reported. Hypotonia and delayed motor milestones and cognitive performance below expectation in comparison to siblings are common. Aggressive behavior, temper tantrums, attention-deficit and hyperactivity disorder may be more common in school-age children. No association has been found between criminality, juvenile delinquency, or sexual orientation and the 47,XYY syndrome. Puberty may be

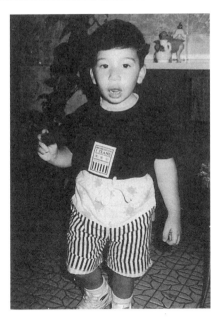

Patient at age 3 years. Note normal stature, long face, long upper lip, and full lower lip. Full-scale IQ was 70. (From James et al., 1995. *Am. J. Med. Genet.* 56:389–392. Copyright © 1995 John Wiley & Sons, Inc. Reprinted by permission of Wiley-Liss, Inc.)

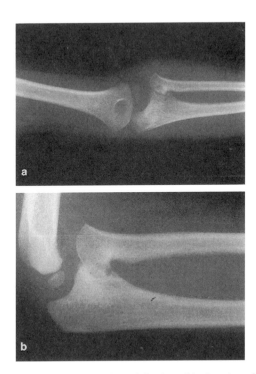

Lateral view of the left elbow in extension (a) and flexion (b) showing deformed radial heads and proximal radioulnar fusion. (From James et al., 1995. *Am. J. Med. Genet.* 56:389–392. Copyright © 1995 John Wiley & Sons, Inc. Reprinted by permission of Wiley-Liss, Inc.)

slightly delayed. Sexual maturation is normal. Persistent severe acne may be noted. Fertility is probably not impaired.

REFERENCES

Borgaonkar DS, Shah SA. 1974. The XYY chromosome male—or syndrome? *Prog. Med. Genet.* 10:135—222.

Hori N, Kato T, Sugimura Y, Tajima K, Tochigi H, Kawamura J. 1988. A male subject with 3 Y chromosomes (48,XYYY): a case report. *J. Urol.* 139:1059–1061.

Hunter H, Quaife R. 1973. A 48,XYYY male: a somatic and psychiatric description. *J. Med. Genet.* 10:80–83.

James C. Robson L, Jackson J, Smith A. 1995. 46,XY/47,XYY/48,XYYY karyotype in a 3-year-old boy ascertained because of radioulnar synostosis. *Am. J. Med. Genet.* 56:389–392.

Linden MG, Bender BG, Robinson A. 1995. Sex chromosome tetrasomy and pentasomy. *Pediatrics* 96:672–682.

Nielsen J, Friedrich U, Zeuthen E. 1971. Stature and weight in boys with the XYY syndrome. *Humangenetik.* 14:66–68.

MONOSOMY X SYNDROME
Turner Syndrome; Ullrich–Turner Syndrome

Monosomy X was recognized by Ford et al. (1958) as a cause of the syndrome of primary gonadal failure and somatic abnormalities described by Turner (1938) and Ullrich (1930). Incidence is approximately 1:2000 female live births. It is estimated that as many as 99% of 45,X conceptuses are lost prenatally. Chromosome 45,X monosomy is found in nearly 20% of first trimester spontaneous pregnancy losses.

MAIN FEATURES: Short stature, hypogonadism, coarctation of the aorta, webbed neck, shield chest

GENERAL CHARACTERISTICS: Short stature is the most consistent feature of Turner syndrome. A number of other somatic, cognitive, and behavioral attributes have been described. The phenotype is highly variable, age-dependent, and influenced by the presence of mosaicism, structural abnormality, and aberrant inactivation patterns of the X chromosome.

Fetuses identified because of posterior cervical cystic hygroma or hydrops in the first or second trimester usually do not survive to term. Newborns with 45,X karyotype typically have normal birth weight and length, webbed neck (pterygium colli), large ears, narrow, highly arched palate, lymphedema of the dorsum of the hands and feet, hyperconvex nails. Congenital heart defect, usually coarctation of the aorta, and horseshoe kidney are found in about 20% of the cases. Shield-chest with hypoplastic, inverted, laterally displaced nipples are commonly observed.

Children and adolescents are most often recognized because of short stature or failure of onset of puberty. Some children may be identified because of learning disability or school failure. Mental retardation is quite rare and when found is often due to the presence of a small ring (X) chromosome that fails to undergo inactivation. Cubitus valgus, short metacarpals, scoliosis, fused vertebrae, cervical rib are occasionally found.

Spontaneous onset of breast development and menstruation can occur particularly in the presence of mosaicism for a normal cell line. Completely normal pubertal development with regular menses is rare.

Neuropsychological studies have shown diffuse right hemisphere dysfunction in children and adolescents with X chromosome monosomy. Full-scale IQ scores are usually in the normal range. Verbal IQ scores tend to be higher than Performance IQ scores.

CLINICAL COURSE: Monosomy X is a highly lethal disorder in fetal life. For live-born girls the life expectancy is nearly normal. Occasional childhood death may be associated with a severe congenital heart defect such as hypoplastic left heart syndrome or total anomalous pulmonary venous return. Adults tend to have a higher incidence of diabetes mellitus, osteoporosis, atherosclerotic heart disease, hypertension, and aortic aneurysm. Pigmented nevi that are commonly found during childhood do not seem to have malignant potential. Keloid formation is more frequent and a factor to consider in cosmetic surgical interventions.

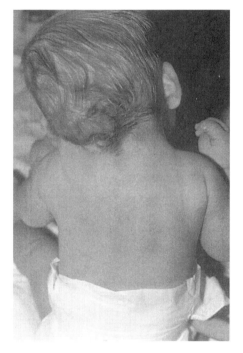

Infant with monosomy X (Turner syndrome) showing webbed neck.

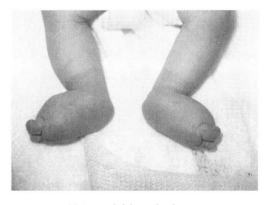

Note pedal lymphedema.

Growth hormone therapy when initiated in children by 9 years of age has been shown to add to the ultimate adult stature. Hormone therapy to initiate and maintain menstrual function is usually required. Osteoporosis in adult women requires attention but the optimal therapy and outcome data are not available.

Naturally occurring pregnancies in women with Turner syndrome are usually associated with mosaicism for a normal cell line. Kaneka et al. (1990) reviewed 138 pregnancies in Turner syndrome. Eighty-two produced live-born infants including 23 with congenital anomalies. Ten of these 23 were due to abnormal chromosomes. In vitro fertilization and implantation of donor eggs can lead to successful pregnancies in women with Turner syndrome.

CYTOGENETICS: About 40% of the patients have monosomy X without a normal cell line identifiable. Isochromosome Xq is found in about 20%. Chromosome 45,X/46,XX mosaicism, deletion of all or part of Xp or Xq, ring (X), and X-autosome translocations are other abnormalities known. A minority of patients have 45,X/46,XY mosaicism. The presence of a Y chromosome increases the risk of gonadoblastoma arising from the dysgenetic gonad.

REFERENCES

American Academy of Pediatrics: Committee on Genetics. 1995. Health supervision for children with Turner syndrome. American Academy of Pediatrics. Committee on Genetics. *Pediatrics* 96:1166–1173.

Hall JG. 1990. "The management of the adult with Turner syndrome: the natural history of Turner syndrome" in Rosenfeld RG, Grumbach M (eds). *Turner Syndrome*. New York: Mercel Dekker, pp. 495–506.

Kaneko N, Kawagoe S, Hiroi M. 1990. Turner's syndrome—review of the literature with reference to a successful pregnancy outcome. *Gynecol. Obstetr. Invest.* 29:81–87.

Kleczkowska A, Kubien E, Fryns JP, Van den Berghe H. 1990. Turner syndrome: the Leuven experience (1965–1989) in 478 patients. I. Patient's age at the time of diagnosis in relation to chromosomal findings. *Genet. Couns.* 1:235–240.

Ross JL, Stefanatos G, Roeltgen D, Kushner H, Cutler GB Jr. 1995. Ullrich-Turner syndrome: neurodevelopmental changes from childhood through adolescence. *Am J. Med. Genet.* 58:74–82.

Turner HH. 1938. A syndrome of infantilism, congenital webbed neck and cubitus valgus. *Endocrinology* 23:566–578.p

Ullrich O. 1930. Uber typische Kombinationsbilder multiples Abartunge. *Zschr. Kinderh.* 49:271–276.

Van Dyke DL, Wiktor A, Palmer CG, Miller DA, Witt M, Babu VR, Worsham MJ, Roberson JR, Weiss L. 1992. Ullrich-Turner syndrome with a small ring X chromosome and presence of mental retardation. *Am. J. Med. Genet.* 43:996–1005.

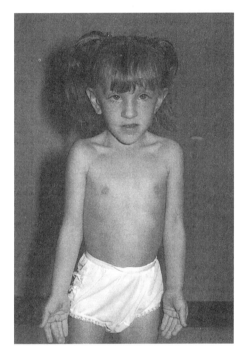

Girl with small ring X variant of Turner syndrome showing triangular face, large pinnae, laterally displaced nipples, and short stature. Her karyotype was 45,X/46,X, +mar, which was later identified to be a small ring (X) with XIST locus deleted.

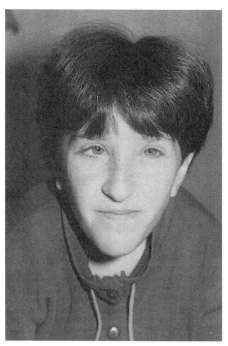 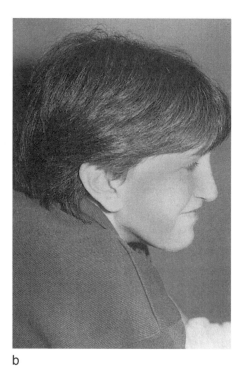

a   b

Patient with small ring X as a young woman with triangular face, severe short stature, and moderate mental retardation (a,b).

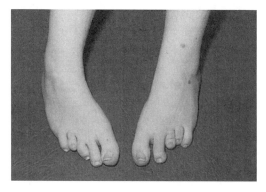

Patient's digital anomalies are apparent.

TETRAPLOIDY AND DIPLOID/TETRAPLOID MIXOPLOIDY

Tetraploidy is a rare cause of congenital malformation. Golbus et al. (1976) described the first live-born patient with tetraploidy. Since then at least 10 cases with tetraploidy and several more with diploid/tetraploid mixoploidy have been reported.

MAIN FEATURES: Intrauterine growth retardation, microcephaly, eye, ear and palatal abnormalities

GENERAL CHARACTERISTICS: Intrauterine growth retardation is common. Placental abnormalities have included thick, large placenta, edematous villi with a paucity of vessels, trophoblastic inclusions, and hydatidiform degeneration. Partial moles are less commonly associated with tetraploidy than with triploidy. Live-born infants with tetraploidy show low birth weight, failure to thrive, and severe psychomotor retardation.

ABNORMALITIES

Craniofacies: Microcephaly and ear anomalies are nearly always present. Microphthalmia and anophthalmia are also common and more so in nonmixoploid cases. Prominent forehead, broad nasal bridge, highly arched or cleft palate with or without cleft lip are common. Micrognathia is recognized in most cases.

Limbs: Hands and feet are described as narrow and long. Long, tapering fingers are particularly impressive in published cases and may be a diagnostically useful sign. Joint contractures as well as positional deformities may be found. Cutaneous syndactyly particularly of the fingers may be less common than in triploid cases.

Other: Congenital heart defects, genitourinary malformations, failure to thrive, poorly developed musculature, and mental retardation are common. Central nervous system malformation and neural tube closure defects have been quite frequently noted. Pigmentary abnormality of the skin has been reported less often in 2n/4n mixoploidy than in 2n/3n patients. One case of a malformed infant with tetraploid cells confined to the bone marrow and only diploid cells in peripheral lymphocytes and skin fibroblasts has been reported.

CLINICAL COURSE: The oldest reported patient is a severely retarded mixoploid 21-year-old woman with multiple malformations, thoracolumbar kyphoscoliosis, spastic tetraplegia, and seizures.

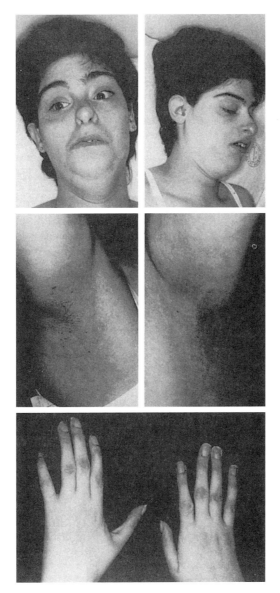

A 21-year-old woman with 2n/4n mixoploidy showing minor facial anomalies, irregular axillary and truncal hyperpigmentation, long, tapered fingers and slender hands. (From Edwards et al., 1994. *Am. J. Med. Genet.* 52:324–330. Copyright © 1994 John Wiley & Sons, Inc. Reprinted by permission of Wiley-Liss, Inc.)

CYTOGENETICS: Tetraploidy is usually due to failure of the first mitotic division in the zygote with resulting karyotypes of 92,XXXX or 92,XXYY. Mixoploidy has a similar origin at a later cell division. Exceptional cases of 3n contribution from the father and haploid maternal contribution have been reported in partial moles. Failure of X-inactivation with absence of a Barr body has been reported in 92,XXXX females. Parental age does not appear to be a factor.

PRENATAL DIAGNOSIS: Tetraploidy has been diagnosed prenatally by analysis of amniotic fluid, fetal blood, and cystic hygroma fluid samples. Tetraploidy in chorionic villi requires confirmatory analysis of amniotic fluid. Maternal serum and amniotic fluid markers such as alpha-fetoprotein and human chorionic gonadotropin have been reported to be abnormal in some but not all cases.

REFERENCES

Aughton DJ, Saal HM, Delach JA, ur Rahman Z, Fisher D. 1988. Diploid/tetraploid mosaicism in a liveborn infant demonstrable only in the bone marrow: case report and literature review. *Clin. Genet.* 33:299–307.

Coe SJ, Kapur R, Luthardt F, Rabinovitch P, Kramer D. 1993. Prenatal diagnosis of tetraploidy: a case report. *Am. J. Med. Genet.* 45:378–382.

Edwards MJ, Park JP, Wurster-Hill DH, Graham JM Jr. 1994. Mixoploidy in humans: two surviving cases of diploid-tetraploid mixoploidy and comparison with diploid-triploid mixoploidy. *Am. J. Med. Genet.* 52:324–330.

Lopez Pajares I, Delicado A, Diaz de Bustamante A, Pellicer A, Pinel I, Pardo M, Martin M. 1990. Tetraploidy in a liveborn infant. *J. Med. Genet.* 27:782–783.

Meiner A, Holland H, Reichenbach H, Horn LC, Faber R, Froster UG. 1998. Tetraploidy in a growth-retarded fetus with a thick placenta. *Prenat. Diagn.* 18:864–865.

Piquet C, Gamerre M, Levy A, Scheiner C, Philip N. 1993. Fetal karyotype from cystic hygroma fluid: diploid/tetraploid mosaicism. *Prenat. Diagn.* 13:770–771.

Shiono H, Azumi J, Fujiwara M, Yamazaki H, Kikuchi K. 1988. Tetraploidy in a 15-month-old girl. *Am. J. Med. Genet.* 29:543–547.

Surti U, Szulman AE, Wagner K, Leppert M, O'Brien SJ. 1986. Tetraploid partial hydatidiform moles: two cases with a triple paternal contribution and a 92,XXXY karyotype. *Hum. Genet.* 72:15–21.

Teyssier M, Gaucherand P, Buenerd A. 1997. Prenatal diagnosis of a tetraploid fetus. *Prenat. Diagn.* 17:474–478.

Wilson GN, Vekemans MJ, Kaplan P. 1988. MCA/MR syndrome in a female infant with tetraploidy mosaicism: review of the human polyploid phenotype. *Am. J. Med. Genet.* 30:953–961.

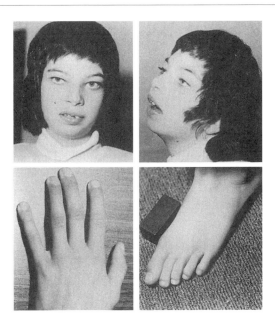

This 11-year-old girl with 2n/4n mixoploidy shows minor facial anomalies, slender hands and feet with long digits. (From Edwards et al., 1994. *Am. J. Med. Genet.* 52:324–330. Copyright © 1994 John Wiley & Sons, Inc. Reprinted by permission of Wiley-Liss, Inc.)

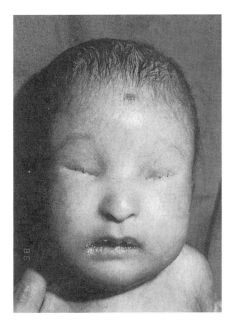

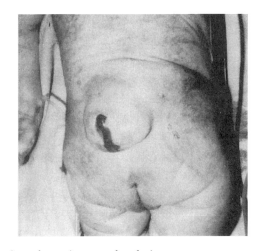

Sacral meningomyelocele is a common finding in tetraploidy. (From Shiono et al., 1988. *Am. J. Med. Genet.* 29:543–547. Copyright © 1988 John Wiley & Sons, Inc. Reprinted by permission of Wiley-Liss, Inc.)

Face of a tetraploid infant. (From Shiono et al., 1988. *Am. J. Med. Genet.* 29:543–547. Copyright © 1988 John Wiley & Sons, Inc. Reprinted by permission of Wiley-Liss, Inc.)

TRIPLOIDY AND DIPLOID/TRIPLOID MIXOPLOIDY

Approximately 1% of all conceptions are estimated to be triploid. Triploidy accounts for about 20% of chromosomally abnormal spontaneous abortions. Fetal loss may be related to hydatidiform degeneration of the placenta. Only a small percentage of triploid conceptions survive to term and this summary of malformations associated with triploidy includes fetuses and live-born infants.

MAIN FEATURES: Intrauterine growth retardation, omphalocele, cleft lip and palate, microphthalmia, syndactyly

ABNORMALITIES

Craniofacies: Large fontanelle, microphthalmia, ocular coloboma, corneal abnormalities, epicanthal folds, and hypertelorism are present in 10–25% of the patients. Low-set, malformed ears are found in 50% of the cases. Cleft lip with or without cleft palate, micrognathia, and microstomia are also common (about 25%). Broad nasal bridge, choanal stenosis, and occasionally arhinia may be seen.

Limbs: One or more of the following limb anomalies are found in virtually all patients with triploidy. In the hands these anomalies include syndactyly, particularly of the third and fourth fingers, single palmar crease, flexion contractures, long fingers, and abnormal dermatoglyphics. Lower limbs show syndactyly, increased space between first and second toes, talipes equinovarus, and rocker-bottom feet. Toenails may be hypoplastic.

Genitourinary: Genitourinary malformations are virtually constant in males. Among these are cryptorchidism, micropenis, bifid scrotum, and ambiguous genitalia. In contrast, external genitalia of females are usually normal.

Organs: Congenital heart defects (septal defects, patent ductus, truncus and dextrocardia), malrotations of the gut, biliary atresia, tracheoesophageal fistula, and renal anomalies are also common.

Other: About 25% of the triploid fetuses and live borns have a central nervous system malformation that may include meningomyelocele, hydrocephaly, agenesis of the corpus callosum, Arnold–Chiari malformation, or Dandy–Walker malformation. Multiple nuclear projections in peripheral neutrophils similar to those found in trisomy 13 and occasionally in trisomy 14 have been described in triploid infants as well.

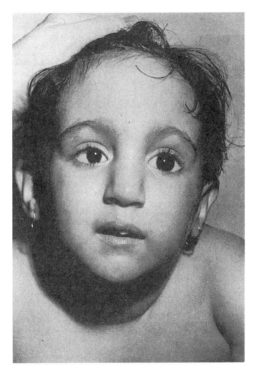

Facial appearance of a girl of 2 years and 1 month with 2n/3n mixoploidy. Note prominent nose with broad nasal bridge and right eye smaller than the left. (From Carakushansky et al., 1994. *Am. J. Med. Genet.* 52:399–401. Copyright © 1994 John Wiley & Sons, Inc. Reprinted by permission of Wiley-Liss, Inc.)

DIPLOID/TRIPLOID MIXOPLOIDY: Only a small number of patients with 2n/3n mixoploidy have been published. The phenotype is milder than triploidy without admixture of a diploid cell line and may go unrecognized in some cases. Most patients with 2n/3n mixoploidy show facial asymmetry or hemihypertrophy, cutaneous pigmentary abnormalities, and mild to moderate developmental delay. Confirming the diagnosis requires chromosomal analysis of skin fibroblasts cultured from punch biopsies of multiple sites.

CLINICAL COURSE: Live-born infants with triploidy usually die in the neonatal period. Diploid/triploid mixoploidy is compatible with survival to adulthood.

CYTOGENETICS: All nonmosaic cases are either 69,XXX (60%) or 69,XXY (40%). No 69,XYY triploids have been found. Fertilization of a normal egg by two separate sperms or by a diploid sperm and failure of extrusion of a polar body are the most common mechanisms of triploidy. Parental age does not appear to be a risk factor. Recurrence risk is low.

REFERENCES

Carakushansky G, Teich E, Ribeiro MG, Horowitz DD, Pellegrini S. 1994. Diploid/triploid mosaicism: further delineation of the phenotype. *Am. J. Med. Genet.* 52:399–401.

Graham JM Jr, Rawnsley EF, Simmons GM, Wurster-Hill DH, Park JP, Marin-Padilla M, Crow HC. 1989. Triploidy: pregnancy complications and clinical findings in seven cases. *Prenat. Diagn.* 9:409–419.

Hassold TJ, Matsuyama A, Newlands IM, Matsuura JS, Jacobs PA, Manuel B, Tsuei J. 1978. A cytogenetic study of spontaneous abortions in Hawaii. *Ann. Hum. Genet.* 41:443–454.

Jacobs PA, Angell RR, Buchanan IM, Hassold TJ, Matsuyama AM, Manuel B. 1978. The origin of human triploids. *Ann. Hum. Genet.* 42:49–57.

Kazazian LC, Baramki TA, Thomas RL. 1989. Triploid fetus: an important consideration in the evaluation of very high maternal serum alpha-fetoprotein. *Prenat. Diagn.* 9:27–30.

McFadden DE, Kalousek DK. 1991. Two different phenotypes of fetuses with chromosomal triploidy: correlation with parental origin of the extra haploid set. *Am. J. Med. Genet.* 38:535–538.

Niebuhr E. 1974. Triploidy in man. Cytogenetical and clinical aspects. *Humangenetik.* 21:103–125.

Niemann-Seyde SC, Rehder H, Zoll B. 1993. A case of full triploidy (69,XXX) of paternal origin with unusually long survival time. *Clin. Genet.* 43:79–82.

Pai GS, Grush OC, Shuman C. 1982. Hematological abnormalities in triploidy. *Am. J. Dis. Child.* 136:367–369.

Sherard J, Beau C, Bove B, Delluea V, Esterly KL, Karesh HJ, Munshi G, Reamer JF, Suazo G, Wilmoth D, Dahlke B, Weiss C, Borgaonkar DS. 1986. Long Survival in a 69,XXY triploid male. *Am. J. Med. Genet.* 25:307–312.

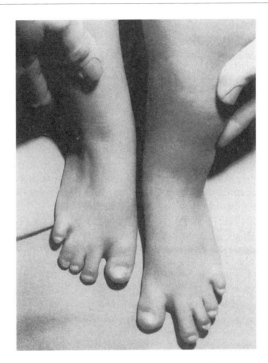

Feet of the patient showing cutaneous syndactyly of toes 3 and 4, increased space between first and second toes, and proximally implanted, short great toes. (From Carakushansky et al., 1994. *Am. J. Med. Genet.* 52:399–401. Copyright © 1994 John Wiley & Sons, Inc. Reprinted by permission of Wiley-Liss, Inc.)

Strobel SL, Brandt JT. 1985. Abnormal hematologic features in a live-born female infant with triploidy. *Arch. Pathol. Lab. Med.* 109:775–777.

Wertelecki W, Graham JM Jr, Sergovich FR. 1976. The clinical syndrome of triploidy. *Obstet. Gynecol.* 47:69–76.

Wulfsberg EA, Wassel WC, Polo CA. 1991. Monozygotic twin girls with diploid/triploid chromosome mosaicism and cutaneous pigmentary dysplasia. *Clin. Genet.* 39:370–375.

Zaragoza MV, Surti U, Redline RW, Millie E, Chakravarti A, Hassold TJ. 2000. Parental origin and phenotype of triploidy in spontaneous abortions: predominance of diandry and association with the partial hydatidiform mole. *Am. J. Hum. Genet.* 66:1807–1820.